THE REBEL DIET
BREAK THE RULES, LOSE THE WEIGHT

MELISSA HERSHBERG, MD

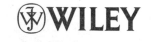

WILEY

John Wiley & Sons Canada, Ltd.

Library and Archives Canada Cataloguing in Publication

Hershberg, Melissa
    The rebel diet : break the rules, lose the weight! / Melissa Hershberg.

Includes bibliographical references and index.
ISBN 978-0-470-73644-9

    1. Reducing diets. 2. Nutrition. 3. Weight loss. I. Title.

RM222.2.H465 2009   613.2'5   C2009-905126-5

Production Credits
Cover Design and Interior Design: Michael Chan
Typesetter: Michael Chan
Printer: Friesens

Editorial Credits
Editor: Leah Fairbank
Project Coordinator: Pauline Ricablanca

John Wiley & Sons Canada, Ltd.
6045 Freemont Blvd.
Mississauga, Ontario
L5R 4J3

Printed in Canada

1 2 3 4 5 FP 14 13 12 11 10

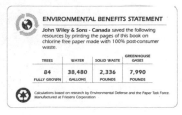

ENVIRONMENTAL BENEFITS STATEMENT
John Wiley & Sons - Canada saved the following resources by printing the pages of this book on chlorine free paper made with 100% post-consumer waste.

TREES	WATER	SOLID WASTE	GREENHOUSE GASES
84	38,480	2,336	7,990
FULLY GROWN	GALLONS	POUNDS	POUNDS

Calculations based on research by Environmental Defense and the Paper Task Force. Manufactured at Friesens Corporation

TABLE OF CONTENTS

Intro   1

Part One: The Rules (that we're totally going to break!)   7
 Rule 1: No Cheating   9
 Rule 2: No Dry Foods   15
 Rule 3: No Sugar   25
 Rule 4: No Carbs   43
 Rule 5: No Fat   57
 Rule 6: No Large Portions   73
 Rule 7: No Booze   81
 Rule 8: No Coffee   89
 Rule 9: No Quitting   97

Part Two: The Goods (that we're going to buy and make)   105
 Fresh Market   107
 Grocery Aisles   123
 Health and Specialty Food Store Items   143

Part Three: The Plan (the route that you're going to take)   147
 Shrink-a-cizing Breakfasts   151
 Skinni-mizing Lunches and Dinners   169
 Rebel-icious Snacks   205
 F&*% Dieting!   213

Acknowledgments   225

About the Author   226

Index   227

DEDICATION

This book is dedicated to my loving parents and grand-parents. Thank you for supporting me and instilling confidence and drive in me, as well as a hardworking, open-minded, occasionally rebellious spirit. And of course, to Ty, for managing to constantly keep me laughing even while driving me crazy.

INTRO

Every woman is a rebel, and usually in wild revolt against herself.
Oscar Wilde

It's the other four-letter word. The D-word. The D-bomb.
DIET.
Why do we hate that word so much?
Hunger. Failure. Rules. Restrictions. Deprivation. Expecta-
tions. Rebound weight-gain. Eating disorders. Strained relationships. Bad foods. Bad moods. Bad breath. Guilt.
There are so many negative associations with the word diet,
it's no wonder that over half the North American population
is overweight. We hate dieting. It's torturous. Tacky. Totally
depressing. And even worse, dieting doesn't seem to work.
The number of diet books, diet experts, and diet products is
increasing each year, yet the rate of obesity keeps rising. So, if
diets make us angry, and hungry, and cranky, and depressed,
and FAT, perhaps it's time to rebel against the diet. Perhaps it's
time to change our approach. Perhaps it's time to shout…

F&*% DIETING!

Yes. That sounds just fine. It has a nice ring to it, don't you
think? Fuck dieting. I like the way that rolls off my tongue.
I like the way saying it makes me feel—rebellious, naughty,
daring, powerful, and *liberated*. Best of all, though, I feel

energized and excited, like I'm holding on to a secret that I'm desperately waiting to tell, all because—get ready for this—I'm about to show you how you can lose weight and improve your nutrition, energy, and health without following the standard diet rules.

I'm going to show you that you can be yourself, live your life, *break the rules*—and still lose weight. You don't have to eat microscopic portions, you don't have to give up bread or chocolate, and you don't have to stop drinking coffee or alcohol if you don't want to. You can make food work for you without being on the same diet you've tried, and hated, and quit a million times before.

Because you're an individual, this book is more than just a "down with diet rules" decree. It's your anti-"one-size-fits-all"-diet bible. And unlike standard diet books, this rebellious approach will give you results. As you'll soon see, *things become so much easier when you stop trying so hard.*

THE REBEL DIET MANIFESTO

Too many people think of dieting as abstinence from their preferred eating habits. It's associated with giving something up: no more coffee, no more alcohol, no more bread, no more pasta, no more dessert, no more meat, and so on and so forth—red lights, stop signs, and "just say no's." Barf. It's as if dieting has become some sort of detox or rehab program, an attempt to learn how to never eat the foods we love again. But this "must be perfect, must never indulge, must always abstain" approach is the problem, and it's why so many diets don't work for the long term. Delicious, convenient foods are all around us, and unless we develop an approach to deal with our cravings and indulge them properly, we'll never achieve lasting success. We'll continue to relapse, we'll continue to gain weight, and worse yet, our metabolisms will be slowed and our food addictions strengthened with each diet cycle. Healthy eating isn't an on-or-off thing; it's not an all-or-nothing endeavor. It's a lifestyle, and until we begin looking at it that way, we'll never succeed.

On the Rebel Diet, you will not be a perfect, abstinent, holier-than-thou dieter. Quite the opposite, in fact. Put simply: You will eat. You will cheat. And you will defeat. Here's how:

Part One: The Rules—that we're totally going to break!

In Part One, we will review the typical diet rules: no fat, no carbs, no booze, yadda yadda. Then you'll learn how to rebel against these rules and still succeed. I'll give you specific strategies and ingenious tips so that you can break the diet rules and still lose weight. In other words, I'm going to teach you how to cheat and get away with it.

Part Two: The Goods—that we're going to buy and make

In Part Two, I will provide you with loads of product recommendations and intelligent shopping ideas, along with practical information on how to find and prepare these "try-it" items. Products are organized in categories just as they would be in your typical grocery store. You can imagine pushing your shopping cart through the store, up and down the various aisles, as I recommend the best choices in each category. You will learn about new, exciting weight-loss and health products such as calorie-free pasta (seriously, it's amazing) and natural, healthy sweeteners that have zero aftertaste and zero calories (like erythritol and FOS). You'll discover new wraps, breads, crackers, and even bagels that taste good and pack in so much fiber that they're virtually calorie- and guilt-free (imagine a whole bagel with the same amount of calories as an apple!). You'll even learn about sweets, treats, and convenience foods that can actually be as good for your waistline as they are for your taste buds. Just incorporating some of these new product ideas into your meals alone will help you on your way to a healthier, leaner life.

Part Three: The Plan—the route that you're going to take (...so that you can throw out your fat pants and let the weight loss begin!)

Armed with the knowledge from Part One and the ingredients from Part Two, you are now ready to embark on the weight-loss plan I have prepared in Part Three. In this final part, I have put together a series of rebel-friendly meal ideas and recipes for breakfast, lunch, dinner, and snacks. There are loads of different options, so you are sure to find something that fits your fancy, whether it's store-bought fare, restaurant selections, or make-it-yourself meals. And I designed this plan to be user-friendly. As a physician, weight-loss coach, and food lover myself, I know what people want—new information that's easy to follow—so that's what I've provided.

Now, the question you've been pondering: how do I know this is going to work? How do I know that you're going to look awesome and get away with cheating? This is how:

A recent study done at Harvard proved what we've known all along: when it comes to losing weight, the actual diet plan—low fat, high fat, low carb, high carb, whatever—doesn't matter. What matters is the amount of calories consumed, plain and simple. Remember, your body is a finely tuned machine, and calories in must equal calories out for your weight to remain stable. Regardless of what plan the subjects of the Harvard study were on, if they consumed 750 calories less than what they were used to, they lost weight. That simple.

Well, duh!

I can't believe that the smarty-pants over at Harvard had to even give this a second thought. I mean, Isaac Newton would be rolling over in his grave! He told us this hundreds of years ago when he stated that calories (units of energy) are never created or destroyed, they just change form. Extra calories taken in from your diet won't just disappear; instead, they'll either be burned off as heat (if you exercise or if you're genetically lucky) or they'll take the form of stored fat (probably on your ass if you're a lady or on your belly if you're a dude). These calories stored on your ass, hips, belly, or extra chin are there for back-up in times of relative famine. For instance, if your body needs 1,500 calories of energy a day to operate and you only feed it 1,000 calories, it will have to grab the extra 500 calories from your fat stores—your hips, thighs, and spare tires. That's why they're there: for times of relative famine. But that's the obvious and easy part. What the study didn't say was how to reduce your caloric intake without feeling deprived and hungry. That's the real story. Well, guess what? I know how (Harvard—call me). It's easy.

You have to eat to maximize nutrient density and minimize caloric density.

Huh, you say? Okay, let me put it in plain English. Basically, you want your food to be rich in nutrients, flavor, mass, and volume without having a lot of calories. When you eat like this the majority of the time, you can afford to eat whatever you want on occasion and still reap the benefits of good health and weight loss. I discussed this in my last book, *The Hershberg Diet*, when I encouraged people to eat high-water foods—foods that fill you up for few calories. Now I'm going to make it even easier by taking even more rules away.

As you'll soon see, losing weight and keeping it off is a snap. You can break the rules, indulge in your favorite foods, and feel great all the while. You'll be throwing out your fat pants in no time.

Get ready, rebels: we're about to eat, cheat, and defeat!

PART ONE

THE RULES...
THAT WE'RE
TOTALLY GOING
TO BREAK!

Rule 1: No cheating.
Rule 2: No dry food.
Rule 3: No sugar.
Rule 4: No carbs.
Rule 5: No fat.
Rule 6: No large portions.
Rule 7: No booze.
Rule 8: No coffee.
Rule 9: No quitting.

Whether you're a serial dieter or you're just concerned about eating healthy, you probably know these rules by heart. You probably mumble them in your sleep as your tummy growls after a less-than-ample dinner, or curse them under your breath as you walk past a tempting, taunting bakery or an impossibly skinny blond-haired bombshell eating an ice cream cone (bitch). But like I said in the intro, they simply don't work. Deprivation and imbalance certainly won't help you be healthy, and they won't help you fit into those skinny jeans any sooner either. They'll only make you miserable, and they'll come back to bite you when your willpower inevitably breaks down. That's why we're kicking these rules out on their asses!

Of course, that doesn't mean you can go nuts. Rebel girls are smart girls, after all. They're informed and in control, and that's what you're going to be by the end of Part One. I'll give you all the info you need to make your own choices, break all the rules, and still look ab fab. So dust off those reading glasses, because we're getting started. Hooray!

NO CHEATING

(Whatever. Catch me if you can!)

Alle Ding sind Gift, und nichts ohn Gift; allein die Dosis macht, daß ein Ding kein Gift ist.

Um, totally! Okay, I don't understand German either, so here's the translation:

All things are poison and nothing is without poison; only the dose permits something not to be poisonous.

As confusing as it sounds, just think about it for a bit. It's terribly meaningful, especially when it applies to food.

This quotation is attributed to Paracelsus, a famous alchemist and physician, and is often paraphrased simply as, "the dose makes the poison." Or, just to really confuse you, it can also mean, "the dose makes the cure." In other words, things that are typically considered bad for you, even toxic, can be absolutely harmless or even beneficial in small doses. On the other hand, things that are considered good for you can actually be detrimental, even deadly, if you consume too much of them. Good can be bad, and bad can be good. And things that are considered healthy and curative are only so if you have enough of them.

IT'S THE DOSE THAT MATTERS! • • • • • • • • • • • • • •
It's impossible to say whether something will have a
negative, positive, or neutral effect on you unless you
know the amount being discussed. If you don't believe
me, consider the following.

The Sun
In moderate doses, it supplies us with energy, heat, light,
vitamin D, and the motivation to drag our bicycles out
of storage and get moving (all good), but if we overdose,
painful sunburns, wrinkles, sunspots, and skin cancer
can result (very bad).

Red Wine
In small doses, such as a glass per day, it provides us
with flavor, comfort, relaxation, antioxidants, even heart
protection (all good), but in large doses, we get brown
teeth, premature aging, bad drunken dance moves, and
increased risk for heart disease, liver disease, and cancer
(nasty). Furthermore, the resveratrol in wine, which has
received a lot of press for its role in slowing down the
aging process, has only proven effective in extremely high
doses. What's an extremely high dose? Well, put it this
way: you'd have to drink about a thousand glasses of wine
every day to get enough resveratrol to make any difference
at all to your "botox clock." And girlfriend, at that dose,
brown teeth would be the least of your problems.

Cyanide
Okay, we all know this is lethal, right? Wrong. Cyanide,
in tiny doses, is actually found in some of the healthiest
foods; like apples, for example. So clearly the dose matters.

Yogurt

We've heard that we should eat yogurt because it contains healthy bacteria—probiotics—that help our guts with digestion and help prevent colon disease. But wait a minute—the average snack-size container of yogurt has hardly enough probiotics to make any difference at all.

Mother-in-Laws

Need I say more? (I love you, Sherrill!)

So why the chemistry lesson? To help you understand why "cheating" on diets and breaking nutrition rules once in a while is okay and even encouraged, and why religiously following the typical diet rules may not be as important as you thought, and can even be detrimental to a sustainable weight loss plan. For diets to be effective and provide the right balance of nutrients, we need variety. To have a healthy, satisfying relationship with food, we need to rebel and allow ourselves to cheat sometimes. And our human nature confirms this time and again by making us obsessively crave things that we think we can't have.

Foods that have received a bad rap—such as bread, red meat, pasta, sweets, fried foods, fatty foods, fast foods, and even some sweeteners, dare I say—are actually okay, and can even be beneficial to weight loss and health…if consumed in the right amounts and in the right way. The dose makes the poison, people! These bad guys don't have to derail a diet program and damage your health. And, as you'll see, they can even prove to be just the thing the doctor ordered to help you lose those extra pounds and keep them off for the long term.

THE TROUBLE WITH DIETS • • • • • • • • • • • • • • • •

As far as I'm concerned, the diet industry has done no favors for the increasing number of North Americans suffering from obesity and related afflictions by labeling everything as either good (approach) or bad (avoid). It's just way too simplistic. I mean, how can something be labeled good or bad if we don't know the dose being discussed? For instance, eating a handful of almonds may be good since it provides antioxidants and healthy, filling fat, protein, and fiber; but on the other hand, gobbling up a whole bag of almonds is a total diet disaster as it provides way too many calories and fat grams. Similarly, enjoying a slice of white bread (the ultimate no-no in most diet books of late) is actually way more waistline- and blood sugar–friendly than munching on four slices of whole grain bread. Doses matter. They can turn good-for-you foods into diet disasters and bad-for-you foods into totally acceptable indulgences. People, people, people—I firmly believe that rigid diet rules have left us fatter, hungrier, and more confused and fearful of food than ever. (It's helped out with food marketing tremendously, though, but that's beside the point.) We have been told that trans fat is the enemy, cholesterol is the enemy, sugar is the enemy, carbs are the enemy, meat is the enemy, fruit is the enemy, and fast, convenient foods are—you guessed it—the enemy. What's left to eat? We can't live on veggies alone. (And aren't they covered with pesticides anyway?) So many of us just give up and say, fuck it, it's too confusing; I'd rather be fat. But it doesn't have to be all or nothing.

We have to stop focusing on playing by the rules day in and day out. We are not perfect little fembots; we are women with cravings, hormone fluctuations, PMS, break-up sessions, make-up sessions, fat days, bloated days, and birthdays. We have lunches to pack, dinner to make, orgasms to fake, and it's all just so exhausting that all we want is a bagel with peanut butter, dammit. On the Rebel Diet, you can have it. And, most importantly, you will still lose weight, improve your health, and feel satisfied and fantastic in the process.

It's our turn to cheat, ladies. And we're gonna get away with it!

The purpose of this book is to review the rules, and then to show you how you can succeed with your weight-loss goals even if you choose to break them on occasion. You will learn about new products that allow you to indulge in ways you never thought possible. These secrets and tricks of the trade aren't just for industry insiders anymore; now you can also learn how to successfully rebel. You'll eat McDonald's; you'll eat bread; you'll eat ice cream; heck, I'll even show you how frozen meals, take out options, and crunchy snacks can totally be incorporated into a healthy lifestyle. This is the Rebel Diet, after all!

Just a quick note, though, for any food addicts out there who are a little afraid of being "unleashed." If you just can't control yourself around certain foods, you don't have to indulge in them just to prove that you're a rebel. While I do encourage you to practice moderation, if you'd rather abstain from certain foods, that is completely your prerogative. As you'll see in the chapters that follow, you will be presented with tips, strategies, recommendations, and options that allow you to eat whatever you want. You will be the one in control.

RULE 2:
NO DRY FOODS

(As if!)

You may think you've never heard this rule before, but I'm willing to bet that you have, at least in some shape or form. Especially if you read my last book, *The Hershberg Diet*.

In *The Hershberg Diet*, I introduced the "fourth macronutrient," and explained that it is the most important factor to consider when eating for weight loss and optimal health. Now that's a pretty loaded statement. So what is this magical substance?

The fourth macronutrient is water. (The other three macronutrients are protein, carbs, and fat, in case you missed that lesson.) But it's not about drinking water, it's about learning how to "eat" water. Foods with the highest water content fill us up for the fewest calories, because water has mass and volume but is calorie-free. Examples of high-water foods are leafy greens and fresh fruits and vegetables (think about how much they reduce down when you cook them—the water evaporates out of them); lean fish, poultry, and meats; egg whites; and lean dairy like yogurt and cottage cheese. These are staple "diet" foods, and for a good reason. They are rich in nutrients, they fill us up—often with valuable protein and fiber as well as water—and they weigh down our stomachs. The average belly needs about 2 to 3 pounds of food each day to feel full. By filling them with water-rich foods, we supply our bellies with the critical mass they need without too many calories.

People have asked me if they can simply eat foods that have little water and just wash them down with a large glass of water to achieve the same effect. Sadly, no. Although it sounds reasonable enough, it just doesn't work. A study done at Penn State showed that when people ate foods high in water, they reduced the number of calories they took in, but when they drank the equivalent amount of water with meals, they did not. The water content of food is the critical factor in reducing our hunger.

So what are dry foods? They're all the over-processed, factory-made carbohydrates, like crackers, cookies, chips, granola bars, and cereals—the munchy foods. When we eat these foods, we take in way more calories than we need because they distort our body's natural built-in mechanisms that make us feel full. Natural foods, the ones that are usually found in European markets or on the periphery of grocery stores, tend to be high in water, with some element of either protein, fat, or fiber. These foods are not designed for shelf life; they're designed for real life. We eat them, they fill our bellies, and then they slowly release sugar into our bloodstream, triggering the appropriate satiation-related hormonal response. Nice, normal, natural. However, when we eat dry, processed carbs loaded with unnatural, artificial ingredients, everything goes out of whack. There's no water to add weight to our stomachs, so we eat more than we intended. The bulky, filling fiber that helps keep sugar levels stable is usually milled out of low-water foods. Worse yet, most of the dry products that line store shelves are packed with high fructose corn syrup (HFCS), which fails to trigger leptin, the hormone that is supposed to help make us feel full. Long story short: dry foods tend to cause overconsumption, binges, and rapid weight gain.

I'm not the first to make this claim about how awesome foods high in water content are, and I won't be the last. For instance, the World Health Organization (WHO) blames the increase in global obesity rates on the increased consumption of energy-dense foods. This, combined with our sedentary lifestyles, has resulted in what the WHO refers to as the "globesity" epidemic. Now WTF are energy-dense foods? They're foods that have lots of energy (i.e., calories) packed into a small space. And how is this accomplished? By creating shelf-stable foods lacking in water, fiber, and protein, and instead replacing these important ingredients with sugar, HFCS, salt, and fat. Think greasy, lard-laden potato chips; crackers, pizza, and fast foods full of chemicals; and teeth-rotting, acne-inducing sugary cereals, chocolate bars, and cookies full of empty, useless calories. (Better yet, don't think about them. They're not even real food, so don't give those fatty bastards the time of day.)

Incidentally, the Okinawa population of Japan, acknowledged to be among the leanest and most long-living communities, has been studied extensively to find out what on earth they're doing so *right*. The one factor that really stands out is their love of low-calorie, high-water foods—otherwise known as low CD foods, which stands for low caloric density foods. They live on fish, miso soup, tofu, sea vegetables, wild yam, and boiled rice; not crackers, chips, cookies, breads, and meat like Westerners. The food they eat has water content and volume, so it takes up lots of room in their stomachs. The food we eat is pretty much the opposite—dry, fatty, and crunchy. As a result, ain't nobody studying our big behinds. (At least not for the right reasons!)

So if I am so confident that high-water foods are the secret to a healthy, skinny-cizing diet, why am I telling you to rebel against this rule? Because there are some dry foods that are extremely healthy and can actually help you lose weight. There are always exceptions to every rule, and I think it's important to mention some foods that, although dry, are very nutritious, not to mention damn good. Furthermore, I know you rebels are totally going to eat dry carbs at some point anyhow, so I might as well give you some tips and tricks on how to consume them with the least damage to your waistline. Here's the rundown on my dry faves.

NUTS AND SEEDS •

Pros: They taste good, add crunch to veggies and salads, are high in vitamins and minerals, and contain healthy omega fatty acids, protein, and fiber.

Cons: Holy shit, are they ever caloric! Most nuts and seeds (such as almonds, brazil nuts, walnuts, cashews, peanuts, pine nuts, and pumpkin seeds) pack about 600 calories per 100 gram (3.5 ounce) serving. For comparison's sake, that's about the same number of calories as in a Big Mac, but half the size weight-wise—100 grams for nuts versus 200 to 225 grams (7 to 8 ounces) for the Big Mac. Yikes. And most of the omega fat in nuts is omega 6, not omega 3 (but more on that in the chapter on fat, on page 57).

My Advice: Eat nuts and seeds sparingly when you're trying to lose weight. Add about 2 to 3 tablespoons for a portion of nuts, which will be about 100 calories, roughly equal to 10 almonds or 8 walnuts. To make it satisfying, don't always rely on nuts alone as a snack or you'll end up eating too many before you're full. Instead, use them as a condiment to add flavor and crunch on top of green beans, salads, fruits, and yogurt. For instance, a pear is a boring snack on its own, but if you slice it up, add just a tad of butter, top it with a tablespoon of slivered almonds and a sprinkle of salt, and then pop it in the microwave for a minute, you end up with a treat that's anything but boring. It's delicious, crunchy, sweet, salty, and filling, and best of all, it gets you full on way fewer calories and fat than the nuts alone. You can also try out two of my favorite nutty products:

Blue Diamond Almond Breeze unsweetened almond milk (chocolate or vanilla)

This is sooo good. It's simply filtered water mixed with crushed almonds, but it's smooth and creamy. One cup has only 40 calories. I drink a glass on its own as a snack, or use it as a base for smoothies or protein shakes. Try it; you'll *love* it!

Bell Plantation PB2 Powdered Peanut Butter

I love peanut butter, but since it's basically oil, sugar, and peanuts, you can imagine that it's pretty high in fat and calories. (Two tablespoons of peanut butter has about 200 calories. Add it to two slices of bread and a tablespoon of jam and you're totaling about 450 calories—wowser!) Even healthy-sounding nut butters like organic almond butter, cashew butter, and walnut butter still have loads of calories, even a few more than regular peanut butter. So I like PB2. It's a dry peanut butter that is just ground-up nuts mixed with a little sugar and salt. You mix 1 tablespoon of water or unsweetened almond milk with 2 tablespoons of dry peanut butter, and voilà: a creamy, delicious spread for one-quarter of the calories of regular peanut butter (about 50 calories for 2 tablespoons). I use it to make a dip for bananas and apples and a peanut sauce for salads and stir-fries, or sometimes I just add it dry into smoothies, shakes, cottage cheese, and plain yogurt to add instant nutty flavor.

DRIED FRUIT •

Pros: It tastes good and contains fiber, antioxidants, and vitamins.

Cons: Since it's dried, it's a concentrated source of calories. Plus, most of the packaged dry fruits contain added sugar and fat. A shocking example is banana chips: a mere 40 gram (1.5 ounce) portion has a whopping 200 calories and 14 grams (0.5 ounces) of fat. Even more shocking is that just a 28 gram (1 ounce) serving (think of the size of a shot glass) of mixed dried fruit has 18 grams (0.6 ounces) of carbs. Most dried fruits are just cleverly disguised, calorie-packed candies.

My Advice: Think carefully before you snack mindlessly on dried fruit, and read the label to make sure there's no added sugar or fat. Use small portions of dried fruits such as raisins to add a little flavor to fresh salads, creamy plain yogurt, or whole grain cereals, but don't overdo it because the calories add up quickly.

If you love the convenience of dried fruit, try this instead:

Freeze-Dried or Bake-Dried Fruit

I'm obsessed with this! Freeze-drying produces a crunchy, dried form of fruit without adding any sugar, salt, or fat. You get the sweetness and crunch without the added calories. The only ingredient is the fruit itself, so, for example, one bag of Sensible Foods 100% Organic Apple Harvest freeze-dried apple chips contains 80 calories (the same as a fresh apple) because the only ingredient is apple. I add them to salads, yogurt, and cottage cheese for crunch, or have them on their own as a snack. And they're a great cereal replacement. In case you were wondering, despite the name, they're not actually frozen or cold; just dry and crunchy.

JERKY •

Pros: It's convenient, satisfying, high in protein, and low in fat (the fat has to be trimmed off before the drying process), and it has a long shelf life.

Cons: Eat a lot of it and you'll be eating too much red meat, sodium, and chemical preservatives.

My Advice: Experiment with jerkies other than beef; try turkey, game, soy, or salmon jerky for something different. Buying jerky fresh from the butcher is nice because it's made from freshly sliced whole muscle meat that's been trimmed of fat, cut into strips, and slowly dried. If you can't get it fresh, here are some brands I really like:

Golden Valley Premium Natural Turkey Jerky

This is one of my faves. It tastes amazing, and it's made without nitrite and from turkeys not raised with hormones. It's a great high-protein snack to have on hand.

The Blue Goose Cattle Company Original Beef Jerky

This is also delish and very satisfying. I keep some at the office just in case I need a high-protein pick-me-up.

CRACKERS •

Pros: They're crunchy, convenient, and good with healthy spreads and dips, and some are low in fat and high in fiber.

Cons: They make you fat *fast* because it's way too easy to eat massive quantities of them. You know the drill: hand in the box, hand in the mouth, fat on the ass, repeat…

My Advice: Don't keep boxes of crackers in the house, even if they say low fat, low sodium, or whole wheat. Chances are you'll eat them mindlessly, and the calories will add up quickly. If you're going to have them in the house, opt for ones that do not contain partially hydrogenated oils and that are high in fiber and low in sodium. Good options are whole wheat matzo or Multifibre Melba Toast, Ryvita, Wasa, and Kavli (thin, crisp crackers), but my absolute favorite is:

GG Scandinavian Bran Crispbreads

These are the best, most satisfying cracker I've ever eaten. One cracker, which is thick and crunchy, has only 12 fiber-packed calories. They are so filling that I need only two or three to satisfy me. I love them with fat-free cream cheese and sliced tomatoes (plus or minus smoked salmon), I love them with a little cheese melted in the microwave (they don't get soggy), I love them with PB2, and I love them with mustard and deli meat. They are a great bread replacement. As you probably can tell, I effing love these crackers, and so will you.

That about covers my favorite dry foods. But while we're on the subject of dry things, I'd like to give a shout-out to dry shampoo. If you haven't tried this invention yet, you should. It's a powder that you massage on your scalp dry, and it soaks up all the grease and leaves you with fabulous-smelling, clean-looking hair. And it adds volume too. So for all of you clever lazy asses who avoid a good sweat because you're worried about having to redo your hair, this is the answer. Massage it on your scalp after a workout and your hair will look better than ever. (FYI—I use Oscar Blandi brand.)

RULE 3:
NO SUGAR

(Yeah right!)

So get this: I'm out for brunch with a girlfriend of mine—an intelligent, accomplished girlfriend—who tells me that she feels sooo much better since cutting sugar out of her diet. She then proceeds to tell me that she thinks her skin is better and her mood is better, and best of all, her pants feel looser. Sounds friggin' fantastic, right? But here's the crazy part: she's telling me this, straight-faced with absolute conviction, while chomping down a breakfast of yogurt, granola, fruit, and honey. Oh, and alongside this "sugar-free" meal, she's sipping on a coffee with milk and Splenda.

What exactly does she think sugar is? She's basically mainlining every type of sugar there is while telling me that she's off the stuff. It's as absurd as a smoker saying they feel much better since kicking the habit…as they puff on a Marlie. However, as little sense as it makes, it highlights two extremely important points:

1. The placebo effect is real and powerful. If people think they are making a positive change, they can actually manifest positive changes and feel better.
2. People are clueless about sugar, and much of what they believe to be true about sugar is sweet nonsense.

Although my dear friend's breakfast was by no means a diet disaster, she most certainly was consuming sugar—and lots of it. Yogurt contains simple sugar in the form of lactose. Granola breaks down quickly to glucose in our bloodstream, not to mention the sucrose (table sugar) that's often added to sweeten it. Fruit contains the simple sugar fructose. And honey contains the sugars fructose and glucose, and actually spikes our blood sugar even higher than granulated sugar itself. And then there's Splenda. Splenda is made up of sucralose, which has been shown to trigger an insulin response in susceptible individuals in much the same way as sugar itself. For someone who is off sugar, that sure seems like a lot of words ending in "ose" to me.

So, sugarbaby, to avoid the mistake my friend made, let's investigate sugar in all its many forms. This section is complex, but it's highly recommended reading because at the end of it, you'll understand how you can eat the sweet stuff without it showing up on your hips the very next day! Now that I have your attention, read and learn.

SUGAR 101 ••••••••••••••••••••••••••••••••

In everyday language, sugar refers to white granulated table sugar (sucrose). Table sugar is the end product of the refining of sugarcane. It tastes sweet (which is good, of course). But it's completely without nutrients (which is bad). When the sugarcane is refined to produce table sugar, the nutrients, such as chromium, manganese, cobalt, copper, zinc, and magnesium, are stripped away. So table sugar is basically calories (4 calories per gram, to be precise) without nutrients, and that's why it sucks big-time from a nutrition perspective. But sugar isn't just

table sugar. In fact, sugar is the building block of all carbohydrates. It can be good and it can be bad, as we'll see.

Varieties of sugar, such as fructose, glucose, and
galactose, can either stand on their own as individual
molecules (monosaccharides), or they can bond with
other sugars to form disaccharides (two sugar molecules), oligosaccharides (three to ten sugar molecules),
and polysaccharides (more than ten sugar molecules).
Lactose (the sugar found in dairy products) and sucrose
are examples of disaccharides. Lactose is created when
glucose and galactose join up, and sucrose is created
when glucose and fructose combine. Kind of cool, but
extremely cool are fructo-oligosaccharides.

Fructo-oligosaccharides (FOS) are formed when
fructose molecules link together. This type of sugar can
be very beneficial for your health *and* your waistline.
Read that sentence again, you rebellious skimmers. I'm
not kidding; this type of *natural* sweetener is actually
good for us and can help us beat diabetes, lower cholesterol, and lose weight. You see, FOS resist breakdown by
our digestive enzymes, so they travel all the way down
to our large bowels, where they act as nutrients for good,
friendly bacteria. This means they have minimal impact
on blood sugar levels and calories, since they're neither
digested nor absorbed. As an added benefit, they're
prebiotics that promote the growth of friendly bacteria
in our colons, which can help promote bowel health.
So this yummy, natural, sweet substance is an excellent
alternative to artificial sweeteners, and I predict it will be
popping up in all sorts of foods quite soon. FOS are naturally extracted from fruits and vegetables such as garlic,
bananas, chicory root, asparagus, leeks, and onions, and

they can also be made commercially by degrading inulin, which isn't bad at all; in fact, just the opposite.

Inulin (which is different than the hormone insulin) is a polysaccharide sugar found together with FOS in many super-healthy fruits, vegetables, and plant foods— Jerusalem artichokes, wild yams, and dandelions, for instance. Like FOS, inulin is not digested by salivary or digestive enzymes, which means that it doesn't cause dental cavities like sugar does, and it contributes very few calories to our diet since it passes through us mostly undigested. The calories don't count—woohoo! And it doesn't increase blood sugar or insulin levels like sugar does—how cool is that? Not as cool, though (unless you live in a frat house, I suppose), is that it can lead to serious gas if you eat too much of it. Oh what the hell, I'll say what I really mean: giant farts. Gross! Although it usually takes more than 5 grams (0.2 ounces) per day to produce a noticeable effect on gas. Just Like Sugar and SweetPerfection, natural sweeteners that recently hit the market have virtually no calories since they're derived from FOS and inulin.

I am willing to bet that, while you may have never heard of inulin, starch and cellulose are polysaccharides that do sound familiar. Starch and cellulose are commonly referred to as complex carbs because the sugar molecules within them are all linked up together in a rather complex way. We used to think that complex carbs were better for us than simple carbs like the — mono-, di-, and oligosaccharides listed above. But we're learning now that isn't necessarily the case. Milk and fruit, for instance—which are simpler carbs—are actually way healthier than some starches, like white bread, white rice, and white potatoes—which are technically—considered complex carbs. This is because most of the complex carbs we consume are so overprocessed that the fiber has been removed, which results in a starch that is very easy to digest and virtually free of nutrients.

Cellulose is the polysaccharide sugar found in plants. Unlike starch, which can go either way health-wise, it's almost always healthy. Even though it consists of many glucose sugar units linked together, we humans can't digest it, so it just passes straight through, adding bulk to our stools and cleaning out our colons. Cellulose is insoluble fiber. It's roughage. It's the stuff found in bran and vegetables. It's awesome for weight loss and regularity.

Just a quick recap: when glucose molecules link together, we get cellulose, i.e., fiber. When fructose molecules link together, we get FOS, which are also fiber, just sweeter tasting. See, it's not so hard to understand, you rebel genius! Let's keep going.

Sugar alcohols (which are not the same thing as those wine coolers that you chugged back in college while gleefully packing on those freshman 15) are another non-digestible sugar; in other words, fiber. They can occur naturally, or they can be made in the lab by tinkering with glucose to add an alcohol group; typically sugar alcohols end in "ol," like xylitol, mannitol, and sorbitol. They taste sweet like sugar, but unlike table sugar, they can't be digested by our intestinal or salivary enzymes, so they don't contribute very many calories to our diet or lead to tooth decay or diabetes. Hurray! But before we jump up and down thinking of all the calories we're going to save, we need to address the horrific gas and bloating that most people, including me, experience after ingesting them. Personally, I stay away because they make me so bloated and gassy that I can't even stand to be around myself. For many people, though, they're quite tolerable, so it depends on the individual. Typically you find sugar alcohols in diabetic products and treats marketed as low carb. There's a new sugar alcohol on the market now, though, that doesn't cause pregnant-looking bloated bellies, liquid farts, or diarrhea, and it's 100 percent natural. And I'm obsessed with it! It's called erythritol.

Erythritol, a naturally occurring sugar alcohol, has all the advantages of the other sugar alcohols except that it doesn't lead to bowel discomfort. Instead of fermenting in our colons, it passes through our small bowel, and then we excrete it unchanged in our urine. In other words, it's natural, we eat it, it tastes sweet, and then we piss it out. This is hugely cool; gigantically fantastic, actually. Erythritol is going to be everywhere soon. You can already find it in individual packets, such as Wholesome Sweeteners Organic Zero, as well as in bags by NOW and Sensato. Truvia is a brand-new natural sweetener that is a combo of erythritol and rebiana from the stevia leaf. It tastes amazing. I love it.

Okay, we're done talking about the good sugars for a while; let's get back to the bad: high fructose corn syrup (HFCS).

High fructose corn syrup, the evil overlord of the nutritional world, is man-made sugar goo as far as I'm concerned. Basically, you take corn syrup, which contains mostly glucose, and then magically alter some of those glucose units to form fructose units. It ends up tasting sweet like table sugar, but it's way cheaper because it's

made from corn (which is easy to grow locally) rather
than sugarcane (which is expensive to import). HFCS
has received a bad rap, and many scientists and nutri-
tionists have associated our rising rates of obesity with
our massive consumption of HFCS. According to figures
from the U.S. Department of Agriculture Economics
Research Service, over the past thirty years, consumption of HFCS has risen from an estimated 0.6 pounds
per person per year to a whopping 73.5 pounds per
person per year. Is it a coincidence that we've also beefed
up during these thirty years? The jury is still out on this.
Personally, I try to avoid HFCS—I'm wary of it, and it's
found in unhealthy products anyhow, like soft drinks,
packaged treats, baked goods, and candies, to name a
few. But remember, the dose makes the poison, so if you
discover you've just consumed it by accident, don't freak
out—it won't instantly make you blow up like a balloon.

And then there's sucralose. It ends in "ose," so we
know it's related to sugar. If you substitute chlorine
atoms—kind of a scary thought, but more on this later—
for the hydrogen atoms on sugar, you get sucralose,
which is indigestible and thus contributes no calories
to our diet. But for many people, it can contribute lots
of—you guessed it—bloating and gas. When you add the
bulking agent maltodextrin, an oligosaccharide sugar, to
sucralose, you get Splenda. Although Splenda is marketed as having zero calories, this isn't really true since
maltodextrin does have some calories—3.75 calories
per gram. Even worse, studies have shown that because
Splenda does contain sugar, it can trigger an insulin
response, which can make some sugar addicts just crave
more and more sugar. Many products on the market

that are labeled "sugar free" or "no sugar added" contain sucralose. (Many of them also contain trans fats, so be on the lookout.)

Phew! As you can see, sugar can mean many things. It can be healthy and good for your diet (FOS, inulin, cellulose, and erythritol, for example), or it can be unhealthy and harmful to your diet (HFCS and excessive table sugar, for example). Sugar is everywhere, so it's pretty darn hard—never mind completely unnecessary— to cut it out entirely from our diets. That's why we're rebelling against this ridiculous rule. Instead of attempting to cut out all sugar, let's be smart with our efforts. Let's eat sugar, but let's chow down on the right kind of sugar, and in the right amounts. Here's my advice and some tricks for you to try out.

FRUITS •

Yes, fruit is mainly sugar, and that's why it's natural to describe it as "sweet like sugar." When I was a kid, my Baba Lilly used to persuade my brother and me to eat fruit by claiming it was "sweet like sugar." (And it was. She added sugar to it secretly. I'm on to you, Baba.) Anyhow, fruit is truly nature's candy. Plus, it's extremely nutritious and packed with colorful cancer-fighting phytochemicals and antioxidants, and loads of fiber and water. And for these reasons, I encourage you to eat fruit. But since it does contain quite a bit of sugar, we need to be smart about our consumption so that we don't spike our insulin levels and acquire a Buddha belly along with diabetes as a result. So here are some tips for eating fruit.

First of all, Baba Lilly may have had to con me into eating fruit by adding sugar, but I'm a grown-up now,

and so are you. Our refined adult taste means we don't
need to add sugar to appreciate fruit. It should be sweet
enough on its own. If you must add something, look
at the sugar substitutes later in this chapter for some
suggestions.

Limit consumption to two to three servings per day.
One serving of fruit is about the size of your hand when
clenched into a fist. So, for example, a medium-sized
apple, two plums, half of a large banana, two tangerines,
one grapefruit, or a cup of berries, grapes, cherries, or
watermelon would all equal one serving.

Avoid fruit juices. I'm sure you've heard this before,
but it's worth repeating. It takes many servings of fruit,
minus their fiber, to make a cup of juice, so you end up
taking in way too much sugar without the fiber, which
results in high blood sugar levels. In fact, when diabetics
go into low sugar shock, we give them orange juice to
quickly raise blood sugar levels. Unless you're in shock,
avoid juice. If you must have it, reduce the amount you
consume by adding just a little bit of it to soda water for
flavor—a virgin mimosa, if you will.

If you have a sensitive stomach, you may want to
eat fruit on its own or before a meal rather than after
it. When you eat fruit after a large meal, it sits in your
stomach and starts to ferment, which causes bloating
and yup, more farts. If you do have fruit with other
foods, try to avoid having it with other high sugar
carbohydrates because the combination could result in
extremely high sugar levels. For instance, a breakfast of
corn flakes, skim milk, and a banana seems innocent
enough, but this meal is very high in sugar and will
likely majorly spike your sugar and insulin levels due to

the lack of any protein or fat to slow absorption. A better choice would be to have half a cup of plain yogurt with half a banana and a few tablespoons of high fiber cereal, oats, or nuts for some crunch. I will give you lots of examples of ways to eat fruit in Part Three.

Try freezing or warming your fruit for a change. Grapes and berries are excellent eaten frozen. A snack of twenty grapes isn't all that satisfying at normal temperature, but when eaten frozen, they're much more satisfying because it takes a long time to eat them, so you really get to savor the sweetness. Also, try warming a cut-up apple or pear sprinkled with cinnamon in the microwave for a minute for a yummy snack.

DAIRY •••••••••••••••••••••••••••••••••••••

Dairy products have fat, carbs (sugar), and protein, and the ratios change depending on the percentage of milk fat present. Cream, butter, and high-fat cheeses are considered fats with little impact on blood sugar, but low-fat milks, yogurts, and cheeses are actually considered carbs, and can have quite a substantial effect on blood sugar. For instance, low-fat frozen yogurts often have eight times the amount of carbs as protein or fat; skim milk has more carbs than protein, and even natural, plain yogurt has 14 grams (0.5 ounces) of carbs compared to only 4 grams (0.15 ounces) of protein. This doesn't mean it's bad; it just means that we have to factor into consideration that lean dairy does affect blood sugar levels. As you can see, dairy is complex and varied in macronutrients, containing fat, protein, and carbs, so it's no wonder that babies can live, grow, and thrive on nothing but mother's milk for months and months.

But, when we combine milk with other foods, especially other sugary carbs like cookies or Froot Loops, it can throw our sugar levels way off balance. Here are some tips for eating dairy intelligently.

Watch out for healthy-sounding, low-fat dairy products with added sugar—stuff like fruity frozen yogurts, puddings, and milkshakes—because they can spike sugar levels very high. Although you can include them in a healthy diet, think of them as significant sources of sugar. Just so you know, a cup of 1% milk has 13 grams of sugar. If you add it to a cup of cereal with a sliced banana and also have a side of OJ, your sugar levels will go through the roof! You might as well have a slice of chocolate cake for breakfast. Speaking of breakfast...

Breakfast is the most important meal because it sets the stage for the rest of your day. If you start off with a super-sugary meal like the one just described, you can bet your ass that you're going to be fighting sugar cravings, hunger pangs, and mood swings all day. Dare I say it, but for most adults, it would actually be better to skip the meal all together than start the day off with one that spikes insulin and sugar. In Part Three, I will give you lots of options for healthy, sugar-stabilizing breakfasts.

Try unsweetened almond milk. This is a staple in my kitchen and office. It's sooo good and it's so good for you. One cup of Blue Diamond Almond Breeze unsweetened vanilla almond milk has only 40 calories, and most of them come from protein and healthy fat. Try this on your cereal to save you some sugar grams.

Add protein powder or ground flax seeds to smoothies, yogurt, and cereal to up the protein and fiber content—both of which act to slow the absorption of sugar into the blood.

Don't be afraid of a little fat in your dairy. I'd rather see a little extra fat than loads of extra sugar. So I'd prefer you put a tablespoon of cream in your coffee rather than spoonfuls of skim milk and sugar. A glug of cream will be less caloric and better for your insulin levels. And I love love love Astro Balkan Style Yogourt. It has 6 percent milk fat, but it is so creamy and filling that you only need a little to feel satisfied, and there's barely any sugar so the calories are pretty low. Did I mention that I love this yogurt? Astro Fat-Free Plain Yogourt is also really good. Sometimes I mix a half cup of the Balkan style with a half cup of the fat-free style—a win–win combo.

SWEETENERS AND SUGAR SUBSTITUTES •••••

One of the easiest improvements you can make to your diet is to limit the amount of table sugar that's added to your food. As I mentioned earlier, it's caloric and nutrientless, the exact opposite of what we want. If you crave something sweet, you can try using one of the more nutritious sweeteners, such as evaporated cane juice, honey, pure maple syrup, and blackstrap molasses. But don't fool yourself into thinking they are any better for weight loss, because they're not. Although they have more nutrients than sugar does, they are just as caloric and spike blood sugar and insulin levels in the same way. To appease your rebellious sweet tooth without derailing your diet, I suggest you follow some of the following tips.

Refine your taste buds, darling. Try to appreciate tastes other than sweet and enjoy food for its subtle flavors and textures. Once you start weaning yourself off sugar, you'll be amazed at how sweet you used to like your food. Sugary cereals, sweet treats, and candy will seem like overkill to your five-star, nose-in-the-air palate.

Use spices, herbs, and extracts for flavor and to bring out the sweetness in foods. Nutmeg, cinnamon, ginger, cardamom, coriander, and vanilla are excellent choices and can make food seem sweeter. Add cinnamon to coffee grinds, apples, and oats and you'll swear they taste sweeter. You can also experiment with almond, banana, coconut, and vanilla extract to add extra punch.

Pancakes and French toast can seem sad and pointless without maple syrup. Not to worry; to keep it sweet but slightly less sinful, dilute your maple syrup with unsweetened almond milk to reduce sugar and calories.

Try agave nectar. This syrupy product is extracted from the juice of a cactus-like plant from Mexico—the same juice that's used to make tequila! But if you, like me, would prefer not to revisit your tequila-shooting days, don't worry; agave nectar won't get you in trouble. It will simply sweeten your foods deliciously and nutritiously without shooting your blood sugar and insulin levels through the roof. This is because it has a high content of inulin and fructose. You can use it to sweeten just about anything; it even dissolves nicely in beverages and homemade salad dressings.

Experiment with some of the new natural, calorie-free sweeteners. Most of them are based on erythritol (a natural sugar alcohol), stevia (a natural sweet herb), fructo-oligosaccharides (FOS), or a combination of all three. My favorite brands are Truvia, Just Like Sugar, and Wholesome Sweeteners Organic Zero packets. But what about Splenda?

If you enjoy the taste of Splenda, I'm not going to force you to give it up. Although there's been a lot of controversy over Splenda, I don't think that it's harmful in moderation. It's pretty hard to get a substance approved by the FDA, and Splenda and sucralose were subjected to years of testing and research, just like any other substance—and they passed. Although there are still conspiracy theorists who doubt the motivations of the FDA and continue to be wary of the composition (specifically the chlorine atoms), studies have shown that all of the chlorine atoms fed to animals as part of a sucralose dose were recovered in the excrement, meaning they peed and pooed it all out. That being said, I still try to use it in moderation because it doesn't provide any nutrients, so there's really no need to OD on the stuff. Two products that I personally love that do contain sucralose, though, are Walden Farms Calorie-Free Maple Syrup (this truly tastes amazing) and Yoplait Source 0% Yogurt cups (a cup has only 35 calories and tastes so good).

DRINKS••••••••••••••••••••••••••••••••••

Most beverages, other than water, milk, coffee, and tea, are basically liquid sugar. Think fruit juices, pop, ice teas, sports drinks, and vitamin drinks, for example. Or if they don't have sugar, then they usually contain some form of artificial sweetener such as aspartame or acesulfame potassium (puke, vomit, gag—I hate the taste of these artificial sweeteners so much, just thinking about them made me throw up a little in my mouth now). If you must have a drink other than water, try these tips:

- Dilute juices and drinks with water, soda water, tea, or Perrier.

- Make your own flavored water by slicing fresh fruits
  and vegetables such as oranges, lemons, limes, and
  cucumbers and adding them to a large pitcher of
  water.
- Add calorie-free True Lemon packets to a bottle of
  water for healthy, summery lemonade.
- Have vegetable juices instead of fruit juices to save
  calories and add nutrients. V8, PC Blue Menu, and
  R.W. Knudsen are great brands. I love them on ice as
  a mid-afternoon snack or a pre-dinner virgin Bloody
  Mary.

DESERTS AND CHOCOLATE · · · · · · · · · · · · · · · · ·

It's pretty obvious that sweets are, duh, packed with
sugar. And that's okay, so long as we recognize this and
choose our portions and indulgences wisely. And I've got
lots of suggestions to help you out.

If you are having mega PMS-style cravings for your
favorite dessert or sweet, sometimes it's best just to give
in and enjoy it. Ignoring cravings will likely make you
feel deprived and sorry for yourself, and the cravings
will only grow stronger as a result. That being said, try
to put limits on these indulgences by only allowing them
occasionally and in small portion sizes. In other words,
if you're craving cheesecake, split a slice with a friend,
don't bake a cake and eat the whole thing when no one
is looking. Trust me, you're not fooling anybody. There's
really no such thing as an anonymous overeater—our
asses give us away.

If you're a chocolate lover, try indulging in chocolates
that aren't as damaging to your waistline and health.
Think of how satisfying and decadent a steamy, creamy
cup of hot chocolate can be. Try Ovaltine, which is

packed with nutrients; 2 tablespoons mixed with hot water and some natural sweetener is great. Add some unsweetened almond milk for extra flavor. Also good on its own is Blue Diamond Almond Breeze unsweetened chocolate almond milk (one cup has 45 calories). If you want to actually bite into your chocolate, try Chocolite Chocolates and Chocolite Finally! bars. They come in awesome chocolaty flavors, and you can satisfy your chocolate craving nicely for a mere 30 calories.

It's better to end your day with a sweet than start it off that way. This advice may come as a surprise, but it's true. When you start your day off with lots of sugar, your insulin spikes and crashes and sets you up for an entire day of sugar cravings, hunger pangs, and irritability. If you end your day with a little something sweet, however, it can serve as a reward and something to look forward to after a day of good eating. Plus, the treat will increase serotonin levels, which can be calming and set the stage for a nice sleep. Don't overindulge, though; too much sugar at night will keep you wired.

Portion-sized desserts such as 100-calorie chocolate bars, ice cream cups, and packaged foods, like Vitalicious 100 Calorie Muffin Tops (finally you can eat a muffin top without developing one of your own—hooray!), can be a great way to indulge in a controlled fashion. Even though they can contain sugar and fat, remember that the dose makes the poison, so a small 100 calorie portion size isn't likely to spike sugar too high. However, be aware that some prepackaged desserts, even healthy-sounding ones such as many of the Weight Watchers snacks, contain trans fats, so read labels and try to avoid ones that have partially hydrogenated oils on the ingredient list.

When you snack, try to balance out the ratio of macro-nutrients—protein, carbs, fat, and water—to get a better insulin response and a lower overall caloric density for the meal. Okay, in plain English, I basically want you to decrease the amount of carbs and calories you eat at one time by adding more water-rich foods as well as either fiber, protein, or fat to slow the release of sugar into your blood. For example, instead of having two large, dry cookies, have one cookie and pair it with a cup of unsweetened almond milk (which is water, fat, protein, and fiber) and some berries (which are mostly water and fiber). I'll give you lots of great ideas for mixing it up in Part Three.

Plan, plan, plan—it's all about planning. You can afford to have awesome sweets so long as you budget your day accordingly. For instance, as you'll see in the meal plans in Part Three, you can have a McDonald's Sundae or half a Dairy Queen Oreo Blizzard because the rest of your day was balanced accordingly. The Rebel Diet is awesome for this reason, if I do say so myself.

So there you have it, sweetheart. Sugar is a complex beast that can be a welcome addition to your healthy life-style so long as you understand the difference between the good kinds and the not-so-good ones. Use the not-so-good ones, like processed, refined carbs, table sugar, and HFCS, in moderation, and allow yourself the occasional indulgence—but don't overdo it or you'll be in fat pants quicker than you can eat a handful of jelly beans. Opt for natural calorie-free sweeteners, such as FOS and erythritol, over artificial ones like aspartame and ace-sulfame potassium. Use nutritious sugars, such as agave nectar, maple syrup, cane juice, and blackstrap molasses, over ones without nutrients like refined sugar—but keep in mind that even the nutritious ones still pack lots of calories, so you can't go overboard. If you follow these basic tips, you'll be looking sexy and svelte in no time. Oh yeah; one more thing: no matter how skinny and healthy you become, liquid farts are never hot, so use good judgment and don't OD on sweeteners, no matter how good they taste.

RULE 4:
NO CARBS

(No way!)

This rule is so crazy it makes me cringe just thinking about it.
First of all, it's dumb…but more on that in a minute. Second
of all, most people who think they're following this rule aren't.
Carbs are everywhere; they're hiding out in fruits, vegetables,
dairy, breads, cereals, pasta, and condiments. They're impossible to avoid. And, more importantly, you *shouldn't* avoid them.

A client came in to see me recently and bragged that he
hadn't eaten a carb in three years. He looked me straight in the
eye and told me this, thinking he was going to impress me. But
here's why I wasn't impressed: 1) he was obviously lying, even if
he didn't know it; 2) after dieting for years, he still didn't
understand the definition of a carb; 3) he was depriving
himself unnecessarily and erroneously, and wasn't reaping any
rewards (after all, he was in to see me for weight-loss help);
and 4) I ain't easy to impress, baby!

Here's what does impress me: understanding the true definition of a carbohydrate, knowing the difference between slow
carbs and fast carbs, understanding the carb–insulin connection, and knowing how to satisfy yourself and reap the nutrition and weight-loss benefits associated with healthy carbs.
(Also, women who can golf and actually enjoy it; people who
can play a musical instrument; marathon runners; people who
have a good sense of direction; anyone who can draw…but
I digress…)

All righty, then. Let's tackle carbs, and then let's cook 'em up and dig in!

Carbohydrates are a category of macronutrient. They have 4 calories per gram, meaning that if you eat 1 gram of carbs, you have just eaten 4 calories. As we discussed in the last chapter, carbs are basically sugar units linked together, but when we refer to carbs in everyday language, we're most often referring to complex carbs: the ones that have lots of sugar molecules linked up, like bread, potatoes, rice, beans, and pasta, so that's what we'll focus on this chapter.

Carbohydrates are our main source of energy, our body's preferred source of fuel. When we eat carbs, they are digested, broken down, and metabolized into glucose. Or more simply, bread, pasta, rice, and cereal turn directly into pure sugar after we wolf them down. This glucose enters our bloodstream and triggers our pancreas to secrete a hormone called insulin. Insulin unlocks the door to our cells, allowing the glucose to get inside. Once inside our cells, the glucose undergoes cellular respiration: basically, our cells breathe in the sugar and pop out adenosine triphosphate (ATP), a form of energy, in return. If our body needs energy, it uses up ATP. If our body doesn't need any more energy—our gas tank is full, so to speak—the glucose is just stored for later use as either fat in our organs and under our skin (jiggle, jiggle) or glycogen in our liver and muscles, or it's given off as heat energy. Because we're such lazy asses these days, with the advent of cars, computers, and ridiculously entertaining reality shows, we don't need that much energy, so surprise, surprise, a lot of that sugar just turns into fat. Boo!

Genetic differences also affect how individuals store their excess energy. Endomorphic body types (think of roundish people who were heavy as kids) tend to store it as fat, mesomorphic types (muscular, athletic builds) tend to store it as glycogen in muscles, and ectomorphs (small-framed types who were really skinny kids) tend to convert to it to heat energy and sweat it off (those lucky bastards).

Carbs have received a bad rap for a few reasons. First, they tend to be caloric. Even though carbs only have 4 calories per gram, the ones that North Americans typically consume are dry, easy to digest, and lacking in fiber. This means that it's easy to take in a lot of grams, and hence a lot of calories, at once. This is an important, albeit confusing, point, so let me elaborate.

Crackers, like Premium Plus or Ritz, for instance, are carbs; they are dry, easily digested (that's why we give them to babies to nibble on), and tend to lack fiber. This means that when we eat a 100 gram (3.5 ounce) portion of crackers (a couple handfuls), we're essentially eating 100 grams of digestible carbohydrate. At 4 calories per gram, this results in a whopping 400 calories. Unless we're really active, we probably don't need that much energy for a snack, so instead of making usable ATP, the calories are probably going to get stored on our body as fat.

Now, let's look at a different carb; a vegetable like spinach, for instance. Unlike the dry, white cracker, spinach has water and fiber (think about how it reduces down to almost nothing when you cook it). When you eat 100 grams of raw spinach (which is a lot, by the way), you are only taking in 15 or so grams (about half an ounce) of actual carb; the rest is water. So you're only eating about 60 calories, versus the cracker's 400 calories for the same portion size. On top of that, the majority of the carbs in spinach are non-digestible fiber, so the calorie count is probably even less since fiber passes through us undigested. The lesson: all carbs are not created equal, so let's stop lumping them together.

A quick note: to eat 100 grams of pure protein (which, like carbs, have 4 calories per gram), you'd have to eat 400 grams (14 ounces)— about half a kilo(!)—of deli turkey. This is because turkey isn't pure protein; it's actually mostly water. (Ever heard that humans are 60 percent water? Well, so are animals.) Unlike munching away mindlessly on a few too many handfuls of crackers, eating 400 grams of turkey is pretty difficult, not to mention expensive. So as you can see, eating complex dry carbs like crackers, breads, and cereals packs on the pounds faster than eating watery carbs like spinach or proteins like turkey, partly because of the sheer amount we're able to consume. Now let's talk about the other factor to consider when eating carbs: the glycemic load.

The portion size, as well as the water, fiber, fat, and protein content of the carb in question, determines its glycemic load. Remember that carbs like beans, breads, and pastas, for example, don't just contain carbs—they can also contain fiber, protein, fat, and water, and this matters when determining the glycemic load. (I'll explain this even further under Rule Six.) The glycemic load is important because it determines how quickly, and to what degree, the sugar from the carbs you eat will enter your blood. If the sugar enters fast and spikes high, this means that insulin will spike high as well. Since insulin is a fat-storing hormone, what do you think happens? We gain weight. Moreover, when sugar and insulin spike, the next thing that happens is that sugar crashes (what goes up must come down!), which results in hunger pangs and severe cravings for more carbs—again, not what you want when trying to lose weight. So, carbs with low glycemic loads can be thought of as slow and steady carbs, while those with high glycemic loads are fast, unbalanced carbs. Slow is good and fast is bad when it comes to carbs. (And sex, of course. Unless you have a headache.)

Let me give you a real life example of this phenom-enon. Many women, at some time in their lives (especially if they become pregnant), have to do something called a 75 gram glucose tolerance test. The test involves drinking 75 grams of pure carbohydrate in the form of a sugary drink. Two hours later, their blood sugar is measured. If it's high, it signals that they are insulin resistant and may be diabetic. But with many women, their sugar ends up being too low (called a hypoglycemic response). See, the sugary drink is a fast carb, so glucose spikes, insulin spikes, and then two hours later, sugar crashes low. When I did this test, this is what happened to me: two to three hours after drinking the sugary drink I felt shaky, starving, confused, irritable, and generally unwell. I didn't know what to do with myself. Lunch was more than an hour away, but there was no way I could wait.

I needed a sugar fix and I needed it bad. I went around the office searching for the most sugary thing I could find, which is very unlike me. I ended up eating two granola bars and a banana—also very unlike me. That made me feel better, temporarily. But two or three hours later, once again I was shaky, sweaty, and ravenous. I went through cycles of sugar highs and lows, and the end result was that I felt hungry all day long, binged on fast carbs, and ended up taking in way more calories that I normally would in a day. This is the danger of fast carbs. This is the vicious yo-yo cycle that so many North Americans fall victim to on a daily basis. Scary shit.

So, am I telling you to banish fast carbs, like candy, crackers, desserts, bread, white potatoes, pasta, and rice, forever? No! God no. But what I am telling you is that eating sugar-spiking fast carbs that have little protein, fiber, or fat content mixed in with them can send you down a slippery slope that tends to lead straight to a giant ass. So here's my advice for approaching some of our favorite carbs.

PASTA ∙∙∙∙∙∙∙∙∙∙∙∙∙∙∙∙∙∙∙∙∙∙∙∙∙∙∙∙∙∙∙∙∙∙∙

I love pasta. But pasta is usually a fast carb. That is why so many people equate eating pasta with gaining weight. So what's a noodle lover to do? Simple: you just have to lower the fast carb portion of the pasta, which can be done in several ways.

Try Dreamfields Pasta. I am in love with this product. The noodles are made with semolina flour and contain inulin, an indigestible carbohydrate that is also a prebiotic (it promotes growth of healthy bacteria in our colon). What this means is that most of the carbs in the pasta aren't even digestible (they're fiber), so they don't release glucose into our blood and therefore do not spike insulin. They're a very slow carb. Initially when I tried this product I was wary. Indigestible carb? Doesn't that mean gas, bloating, and diarrhea? But amazingly it didn't. And it tastes, looks, and cooks exactly like pasta. The noodles come in linguine, spaghetti, and lasagna shapes. About a cup and a half cooked makes a good portion size.

Use whole wheat, high-fiber pastas over white pastas whenever you can. You can also try noodles made from quinoa, flax, and soybean. Catelli and Nutrition Kitchen are good brands.

White flour pasta is not terrible, so don't feel too bad if you want to indulge once in a while. At least it has water content (the noodles swell up and absorb water when you cook them in water), so they're not dry, which is a plus. However, since white pasta lacks protein and fiber, it can spike blood sugar and insulin levels, making you more likely to overeat. If you're having white pasta, watch the portion size. Have an appetizer size or just a small amount on your plate (half a cup cooked) mixed with fibrous vegetables, and avoid cream sauces.

Shirataki noodles are by far the best new product I've come across of late. They are awesome; fantastic; a dieter's dream. These are truly amazing: they look like noodles and work like noodles, but get this: they have *zero* calories. Nope, not a typo. I know it's a real noodle-scratcher, but believe it or not, these noodles have no calories because they're made from water and a little soluble fiber (yam flour). You can buy them plain at most Asian grocery stores (I love the Shirakiku brand), or House Foods makes a fantastic variety that has some

tofu mixed in for texture. A whole bag of House Foods
Tofu Shirataki Noodles has only 40 calories, and they
are unbelievably good and easy to cook with. I use them
anywhere I would pasta, but they're especially good in
stir-fries, soups, and creamy "pasta" dishes. I've provided
lots of suggestions for cooking with them in the recipe
section. These noodles are great on their own, but they're
also fantastic added to rice and whole wheat pasta to
expand the portion size without expanding the calories.
My clients love these noodles, even my Italian clients!

BREAD

I've never met anyone who didn't like bread. It smells
amazing, tastes amazing, has fantastic texture, and is so
cheap and easy to work with. Bread rocks. But bread is
many a dieter's nemesis. We stand at the kitchen counter
tearing off piece after piece and spread butter, peanut
butter, mayo, whatever on it to our heart's content. It calls
to us at restaurants, bakeries, and coffee shops. It's divine.
But we can't have it if we want to be slim and healthy...or
can we? Of course we can! We're rebels; we can do what
we want and get away with it. And I'll tell you how.

Look for breads with low yeast content, because yeast
equals sugar. The flatter the bread, the less yeast it has. So
fluffy white breads are not your best option. In Part Two,
I'll give you some examples of my favorite bread picks.
For instance, look for breads that have high fiber and
are sliced thinly. Weight Watchers 100% Whole Wheat
Sliced Bread is a good example. Two slices have fewer
than 100 calories.

Experiment with tortillas. Tortillas, especially high-
fiber whole grain ones, can be excellent to eat when

you're trying to lose weight. La Tortilla Factory makes a large, delicious tortilla that has only 100 calories. I use it as a base for pizzas and quesadillas, and as a wrap for lunches.

If you love bagels, try Baker's Deluxe High Fibre Bagels. They have only 90 calories in a whole bagel, which is about a third as many calories as in a regular bagel. Plus, they're seriously filling. Try one toasted with light strawberry cream cheese for a delicious, bready breakfast.

Skip the bread basket at restaurants. You're usually starving when you sit down at the table, so you end up eating more bread than you intended. Plus, the bread they serve, although tasty, is usually the worst kind for you— warm, buttery, salty, fluffy, and delicious. Grr. My trick is to order a virgin Bloody Mary or virgin Bloody Caesar if I'm really hungry when I get to the restaurant. I can eat the celery and olives it comes with, and the fiber in it fills me up so I can resist the bread. Or just ask your server to not bring bread if you don't trust your willpower. (If he or she does by accident, either send it back or "accidentally" spill water on it so you don't eat it. Although you probably shouldn't do that if you're on a first date.)

POTATOES, RICE, AND SQUASH • • • • • • • • • • • • •

This tip really is important: opt for sweet potatoes over white potatoes. White potatoes are very high on the glycemic index, but sweet potatoes aren't. Plus, they're super flavorful, so you don't even need to add any toppings to them, and for a filling side dish, they're totally low on the calorie scale (one medium-sized sweet potato has only 120 calories or so; that's about the same as an apple).

Experiment with potato skins. Bake a potato, scoop out most of it, and stuff in some vegetables or salsa or a wedge of Laughing Cow Light Cheese—or hell, why not veggies and cheese?—for a very satisfying high-fiber, low-calorie side dish.

Rice is a great side dish that can and should be part of a healthy weight loss plan—provided you watch portion sizes, fattening additives, and the overall gylcemic load. Good ways to do this are to choose brown and basmati over white rice, and to accompany the rice with vegetables and lean protein to lower the meal's glycemic load. Think of a half cup of cooked brown rice as the equivalent to one slice of whole grain bread—both are about 100 calories, but the rice has far more water, volume, and mass, so it's more filling. Try making a rice "sandwich" for lunch or dinner: put a half cup cooked brown rice on the bottom of your bowl or plate; scoop steamed, seasoned vegetables and lean protein (like deli meat, fish, scrambled egg whites, chicken, or shrimp) in the middle; and put another half cup of brown rice on top. Yum! So good for lunch or dinner—filling, delicious, and nutritious.

Squash rocks for weight loss. Spaghetti squash has about 40 calories per cup when cooked, and butternut squash has about 60 calories per cup cooked. Do you know how low that is, people? That's like half-a-banana low, five-nuts low, burned-off-with-seven-minutes-of-walking low. In other words, you should go buy some now and experiment with it. I love the taste of squash, and it makes a great side dish. Toss diced butternut squash with a little olive oil and some kosher salt, bake in the oven at 400 degrees Fahrenheit for 45 minutes, and you have delicious, nutritious fries!

CEREAL ●

Cereal, the innocent-sounding food we remember so
fondly from childhood, can wreak havoc on diets if
you're not careful. We give cereal to kids because it's
fortified with vitamins and minerals (good insurance if
they skip their fruits, veggies, and meats, as they often
do) and because they'll actually eat a decent portion of
it. Problem is, if kids can eat a bowl of the stuff, you can
bet your booty that we grown-ups can eat three bowls
no problem. And we do. Admit it: how many times have
you stuck your hand into that cereal box over and over
again? How many times do you pour just a little more
cereal out of the box to sop up the extra milk, and then
add more milk to moisten the extra cereal? Cereal is
dangerous, but it can also be healthy and an easy meal in
minutes. So if you're going to indulge, follow this advice.

Choose varieties that fill up your bowl for the fewest calories, like ones that are puffed full of air. After all,
air takes up space but has no calories. I love Nature's
Path Kamut Puffs. One full cup has only 50 calories (for
comparison's sake, one cup of bran flakes with raisins has
190 calories).

Avoid sugary cereals and ones that contain dried fruit.
They pack a ton of sugar and will throw your hormones
right out of whack, starting the cycle of sugar highs and
lows for the day. If you want a sweet taste, add one of the
natural, low-calorie sweeteners listed in the previous chapter, or add in a bag of Sensible Foods Crunch Dried Fruit.

Another great way to lower the glycemic load of your
favorite cereal is to simply eat less of it. Use it as a condiment, rather than the main focus, by adding just a few
tablespoons atop yogurt or cottage cheese.

BEANS AND LEGUMES • • • • • • • • • • • • • • • • • • •

Here's an example of an über-healthy carb that packs protein as well as fiber. As a result, beans and legumes are low on the glycemic index and provide an awesome balance of nutrients. Most beans and legumes, such as chickpeas, soy beans, lentils, kidney beans, and green peas, have approximately 100 calories for a half cup cooked, about the same as a half cup of brown rice or whole wheat pasta, but they're much higher in protein and fiber. In addition to keeping an eye on portions, here's some stuff you should think about when eating your beans.

Because beans and legumes do contain protein, they can make a fab vegetarian substitute for meats and fish. You must keep in mind, however, that unlike meats and fish, legumes pack quite a bit of carbs. So be careful to keep an eye on the carbs in the rest of your meal. Pair them up with less carby foods, like salad greens, veg-etables, shirataki noodles, and soups, rather than heavy starch hitters like heaps of rice.

Sauces matter. For instance, if you order chickpea or lentil dishes at some Indian restaurants, the calories skyrocket because the sauces can be full of butter and cream. Rather than curry, opt for dal when you eat at Indian restaurants because it's typically just lentils and spices with a little oil or clarified butter. (You can even ask them to go light on the oil or butter to make it even healthier).

Be aware that bean salads and green salads are very different entities. Bean salads can have soaring calorie counts, as they often pack a cup's worth of beans at least, as well as oil and rice. Green salads, on the other hand, are very low in calories because they're mostly leafy greens and vegetables. You're better off ordering a green salad and then adding beans yourself so you can control how much oil and beans you add. That's the way to go.

Bean spreads can be a great way to add protein and fiber to your breads. Try two tablespoons of hummus on a piece of whole grain bread with some sliced tomatoes and basil for a yummy snack. Or make a quick lunch by stuffing half of a whole wheat pita with two tablespoons of hummus, salsa, cucumbers, and alfalfa sprouts. Give Guiltless Gourmet Fat Free Black Bean Dip a try; at 40 calories per two tablespoons, it really is guiltless!

Now that we've exposed carbs for what they really are—pretty darn good sources of nutrients when eaten correctly and in the right amounts—I hope you're able to appreciate and embrace them as part of your Rebel Diet. When you cut carbs drastically one day and then bring them back the next, you'll always feel like you're fighting water retention, because you are. Cutting carbs for a day causes you to dehydrate a bit, yes; but when you inevitably add them back into your diet—as you do on vacation or at a party—you'll bloat up faster than a zit on your chin the night before your wedding. When you eat carbs steadily, though, you don't have to worry about shrinking and ballooning on a daily basis. Best of all, you'll have so many more choices at meal time. Skip over to Parts Two and Three for a minute if you need proof. But then flip back pronto, because we're about to discuss the F word.

NO FAT

(Fat chance!)

Even I've said it before: you are what you eat. However, this doesn't necessarily mean that if you eat fat, you'll become fat. Let's not be so literal, people. After all, if you eat sugar, are you sweet? Not necessarily. Trust me; I've known many a sugar-loving bitch in my time. I am one sometimes! So now that we've cleared that up, let's chat fat.

Fat. It can be white, yellow, and brown; good for us and bad for us; beautiful and fugly. And it can be found in many forms: saturated, monounsaturated, polyunsaturated, and trans. It's complicated, so let me melt it down for you.

White fat is the subcutaneous fat that is found beneath your skin. It's the jiggly, grabbable, and often dimply stuff that everyone is so desperately trying to get rid of. It's the fat that prevents our muscles from showing through, the fat that hides our six-pack no matter how many crunches we do. It's the fat removed by liposuction. Although unsightly, subcutaneous fat is often harmless. It cushions and protects our bodies, it adds curves and shape, it acts as an energy reservoir, and it keeps us warm and insulated.

Genetics determine how much subcutaneous fat a person can store. Some people have a great capacity to store sub-cutaneous fat (endomorphic body types, more typical of people from cold climates), while others store only a relatively small amount no matter how much they eat (ectomorphic body types, more typical of people originating from hot, tropical climates). When our subcutaneous fat stores become too great for our own body's particular liking, that's when the trouble starts.

When we gain too much weight, we overwhelm our fat cells. Because we have a relatively stable number of fat cells, we simply store more and more in each cell, causing them to get bigger and bigger until—pop—the contents spill into the blood and pollute it. Fat cell contents include hormones, triglycerides, and toxins, and when they spill into our blood they cause all sorts of problems, ranging from increased estrogen levels (which increases risk for breast cancer and, um, man boobs), elevated triglycerides (which increases risk for heart disease and stroke), and general inflammation in the body. On top of that, when subcutaneous fat stores are overwhelmed, the body starts to store fat in more dangerous places, such as our liver, pancreas, blood vessels and peritoneal cavity. This fat is known as visceral fat, and it's downright dangerous. Visceral fat is yellow fat. It tends to cause our bellies to look swollen and hard rather than jiggly and soft (think of pregnant-looking men with skinny legs and bums—that's the look of visceral fat).

Visceral fat impairs the functioning of our vital internal organs. In fact, it is estimated that fatty liver disease, the result of storing fat in our liver, will soon overtake alcohol as the leading cause of fatal liver disease. There's also a theory that visceral fat sends signals to the liver to produce more glucose and reduce the body's sensitivity to insulin, causing diabetes.

To recap, then: gaining too much fat is dangerous because it causes hormones and toxins to accumulate in

the blood, and it causes serious damage to our internal
organs.

Here are some signs that your level of body fat may be
too high for your body's liking:

- Your doctor has told you that you have fatty liver or
  elevated liver enzymes.
- You have increased abdominal circumference (men
  greater than 40 inches, women greater than 35
  inches).
- Where you store fat has changed, and you are now
  noticing more and more fat around your waist.
- Your HDL (good cholesterol) is low.
- Your level of triglycerides (fat in your bloodstream) is
  high.
- You have elevated blood sugar, pre-diabetes, or
  diabetes.
- You feel bloated in your abdomen.
- You have stick legs, a tiny bum, and a belly like Santa
  Claus.
- You have gout.

Here's the good news. While subcutaneous fat can be
difficult to lose, visceral fat is easy to lose because our
bodies desperately want to get rid of this stuff. This is
why men, who tend to have less of a capacity to store
subcutaneous fat and therefore start to store visceral fat
earlier, tend to lose weight fastest on diets (bastards!).
They lose visceral fat and their pregnant-looking, swollen bellies shrink. Weight loss is incredibly important for
men because as they lose this visceral fat, their risk for
heart disease, stroke, and diabetes goes way down.

Women, especially premenopausal women, tend to be able to store more subcutaneous, benign fat on the buttocks, hips, legs, bellies, and breasts before their bodies begin making visceral fat. That means muffin tops, thunder thighs, and lots of junk in the trunk. Aren't we lucky? I guess so, because this is why women tend to have lower rates of heart disease than men. Unfortunately, this ripply, jiggly body fat can be difficult to lose, as many gals know all too well. It's a good thing and a bad thing. A good thing because the doors to the fat cells open easily to let more and more subcutaneous fat in, preventing it from becoming dangerous visceral fat. But it's a bad thing because: 1) few women want any more fat on their asses, and 2) the fat cells' doors don't open as easily on the way out. So it's easy for fat to get in, but a bitch to get out. Eventually, though, it can be done, so don't give up.

What about HDL and LDL, those letters your doctor keeps blabbing about to you? Those are just types of fat carriers in the blood; good and bad, respectively. HDL picks up greasy, yellow fat in our blood vessels and carries it back to our liver to get rid of it. So HDL is good cholesterol that helps keep our arteries clean (think "H" for healthy). You want this stuff. LDL, on the other hand, takes cholesterol from our liver and brings it to our arteries to store and accumulate. This sucks because this yellow, greasy fat causes blockages that can lead to heart attack and stroke (think "L" for lousy).

Deep breath. Stretch. Let's continue. Only a couple more fats to deal with before I tell you about all the yummy fatty foods you actually get to eat. (And all the nasty fat you can't. Well, maybe sometimes. We are rebels, after all!)

We've discussed white fat and yellow fat, so let's move on to the brown stuff. Brown fat is good. In fact, it's great; we *want* brown fat. But we can't have it. You see, brown fat is a calorie-burning powerhouse. It has tons of mitochondria and is excellent at turning the food we eat into heat rather than fuel or white fat. In other words, the more brown fat we have, the skinnier we'll be because we're burning more calories. Babies are born with lots of brown fat, often found on the back between the shoulder blades. It's there to keep them warm because it produces lots of heat. As we get older, though, we lose our brown fat, and it becomes harder and harder to keep slim. But certain people retain more brown fat than others. Those genetic lucky ducks have an easier time staying thin because so much of the energy they consume is burned off as heat rather than stored as fat. Maybe they sweat a lot? In fact, they likely do. Overweight people sweat at rest because they have too much fat—too much insulation. Skinny people sweat at rest because they have more heat-producing, calorie-burning brown fat. Unfair? Yes. But in evolutionary terms those skinny, sweaty bitches have the survival disadvantage because they'd die off in times of famine. Still annoying, though. Maybe one day soon they'll figure out how to do brown fat transplants? A girl can dream.

Okay, let's talk about food now.

When we look at the fat in food, it all comes down to the science of double bonds. When a fat has no double bonds between the atoms in its chemical structure, we call it a saturated fat. Saturated fats, like the fat in cream, cheese, egg yolks, and meat, tend to be fairly solid at room temperature. So, saturated fats = no double bonds

= solid (think butter, cheese, and marbling in meat). When a fat does have double bonds in its structure, though, we call it unsaturated.

With unsaturated fats, what matters is how many double bonds are present, where they are, and in what form those double bonds are in: cis or trans. Mono-unsaturated fats, like the kind in olive oil, have one double bond that's in cis form. Polyunsaturated fats, like the kind found in plant foods such as nuts, seeds, soy, algae, and the fish that eat them (salmon, for instance), have many double bonds that are in cis form. If the first double bond is in the third carbon position, we call it an omega 3 fat; if the first double bond is in the sixth carbon position, we call it an omega 6 fat. We must get omega fats from our diet because our bodies can't make them, so they're called essential fatty acids (EFAs). Transunsaturated fats, aka trans fats, also have double bonds...but they've been partially hydrogenated, which changes the configuration of the double bond from cis to trans.

I know it's all a little complicated and dull, but that last point is important because *it ruins everything!*

Some trans fats are found naturally in trace amounts in beef and cream. But the vast majority of trans fats have been created by the food processing industry by partially hydrogenating vegetable oils. These partially hydrogenated oils—trans unsaturated fats—are most commonly found in fast foods, baked goods, snack foods, and fried foods. Why? Because hydrogenated oils are fabulous for extending the shelf life of products and for decreasing the need for refrigeration. They're also easy and cheap to work with. So a dream come true, right?

Yeah right. Trans fats are a freaking nightmare. They clog up our arteries and wreak havoc on our health. Saturated fats and unsaturated fats are useful; we need them to function. Trans fats are not.

Since there are so many different types of fat, it's unfair to lump them all in the same category and declare that fat is bad and we should run screaming from it. Instead, we have to look at each individual fat, the quantity we're using, how we're using it, and what it's combined with.

TRANS FATS •

Trans fat is bad. Avoid it. Don't freak out if you eat it by accident or on very rare occasions—remember, the dose makes the poison—but I try to stay away from this non-nutritious, unhealthy fat whenever I can. A good rule of thumb is to avoid foods that contain the phrase "partially hydrogenated oil" in the ingredient list. This means there's trans fat involved. Even though the label may say zero trans fats, if it says partially hydrogenated oil on the ingredient list, it's there. Zero doesn't really mean zero. A label can report zero trans fats if there's less than 0.5 grams in the product, so always check the ingredient list. Fractionated oil, however, is not the same as partially hydrogenated oil and is not trans fat.

Trans fats tend to hide out in foods that have shelf lives (a shelf life means it'll shorten our lives, people). Even some foods that seem healthy contain trans fats, so you really need to watch out. For instance, I was recently looking at the ingredient list on some Weight Watchers packaged desserts, and was surprised to discover that they too contained trans fats. Nutrition bars, granola bars, 100 calorie snack packs, and even foods marketed as ultra low fat, such as Cool Whip 95% Fat Free, can have trans fats, so please look at the ingredients before you buy. The products I have selected for you in the grocery list do not contain trans fats.

SATURATED FATS •

Saturated fat has been called good, bad, and everything in between. Near the end of the twentieth century, saturated fat developed quite a bad rap and was blamed for everything from heart disease to cancer. We were encouraged to avoid foods that contained a lot of saturated fat. Most saturated fat is found in animal foods, such as dairy, meat, and eggs, so people began to stay away from animal foods, but they did it all wrong. They took the advice as a license to eat way too many non-nutritious, low fiber, fat-free carbs and candies (sugary cereals, white pasta, potatoes, and bread), and they gave up butter and replaced it with cheap margarine, partially hydrogenated oils, and omega 6 oils such as corn, safflower, and sunflower. As we are now all too aware, this did not turn out well—obesity, diabetes, and heart disease rates sky-rocketed, and we're now fatter than ever. Saturated fat was not the disease-causing enemy it had been reputed to be. That's not to say that it's excellent for us, just that it's not always dangerous. It can even be beneficial if consumed in proper amounts.

Our bodies need some saturated fat in our diets, and that's why so many natural foods have it, from breast milk to meat to nuts to fish. Saturated fats are important for cell membranes, cell messaging, hormone production, and transport of vitamins such as A, D, E, and K.

However, like most things in life, too much of a good
thing can turn ugly. So when it comes to eating foods
with saturated fat, we should choose nutrient-rich varieties, and we should limit the dose by choosing reduced-
fat foods, when possible, and watching portion sizes. I'll
give you some tips.

Buy organic meats, dairy, and eggs whenever possible.
Hormones, toxins, and pesticides hang out in fat, so it's
best to buy organic varieties that were raised without
pesticides, hormones, or antibiotics.

Limit red meat to no more than one or two servings
per week. Choose lean varieties of beef, lamb, pork, and
veal such as tenderloin, sirloin, filet mignon, and lean
ground varieties. Try to buy organic and grass-fed meat
whenever possible. Trim visible fat off the meat and use
lower fat cooking methods such as boiling, broiling, baking, and barbecuing. Consume leaner meats more often,
such as chicken, turkey, and game, as they have ample
protein to keep you full and the saturated fat content is
quite low.

Use egg whites instead of whole eggs to save your fat
calories. Although the egg yolk contains healthy nutrients such as choline, it is caloric. The yolk is fat (60
calories); the white is water and protein (15 calories). So
when making omelets or egg salad, you may want to use
one whole egg plus two egg whites to save yourself the
calories. For egg wash, use two egg whites mixed with
skim milk or buttermilk. I have an easy recipe for French
toast using this trick, see page 163. And buy organic eggs
containing omega 3 whenever you can. These eggs come
from chickens that were fed flax seeds. Flax seeds are
high in omega 3. It's the circle of life, baby.

Choose lean dairy products, but be wary of those low-fat or fat-free products that have been loaded up with sugar instead. I'd rather see you eat a high-fat plain yogurt than one with less fat that's been sweetened with heaps of sugar. The high-fat plain yogurt will be thick, satisfying, and filling, but the low-fat one will be less filling and more likely to trigger a sugar craving. I often buy plain yogurt and sweeten it myself using natural calorie-free sweeteners such as erythritol, oligofructose, or stevia (lots of good suggestions are on page 132). Or I add a little bit of fresh fruit or half a bag of freeze-dried fruit. My favorite yogurt by far is Astro Original Balkan Style Natural Yogourt; it has 6 percent milk fat (saturated), but has practically no sugar and zero sweetener. It has only 90 calories in a half cup and fills me up way more than other lower fat varieties. Yum! I'm going to have a bowl right now.

Opt for light or part-skim cheeses and be mindful of portion size. Reduced-fat sour cream, cream cheese, cottage cheese, plain yogurt, and skim or part-skim cheeses are great to have in the kitchen.

Try cooking with virgin coconut oil. It's a saturated fat, but it has medium chain fatty acids that withstand high temperatures without oxidizing and creating evil free radicals.

UNSATURATED FATS •

At around the same time saturated fats were being touted as the enemy, unsaturated fats were being praised, appearing everywhere from packaged, shelved, baked, and processed foods to salad dressings and even baby foods. The problem, though, was that there wasn't enough of a distinction being made between the different types of unsaturated fats: mono, trans, omega 6, and omega 3. So people used the cheapest and easiest-to-work-with ones: the omega 6 fats (corn, soybean, vegetable, cottonseed, safflower, and sunflower oils) and the trans fats (partially hydrogenated vegetable oils, margarine, and shortening). As is the case with many things in life, if it comes cheap and easy, *run*— it's probably too good to be true. And it was. Turns out that if we eat too much omega 6, the ratio of fats inside of us gets all out of whack and we increase our risk for blood clots, inflammation, heart attack, stroke, cancer, and depression. So what's the answer? We need to decrease our omega 6 oils and trans fats and increase our omega 3 oils and monounsaturated fats to get the balance back in favor of health.

Experiment with flax, hemp, and salba. These plant foods are high in omega 3 fatty acids as well as protein and fiber. Grind flax seeds (or buy them pre-ground) and use a tablespoon on top of yogurt (FYI: a tablespoon of ground flax seeds has 30 calories). Try salba seeds and sprinkle them on yogurt or dissolve them in your shake. Or experiment with hemp seeds, adding a tablespoon to your morning smoothie; this alone will add 5 grams (0.2 ounces) of protein and loads of omega 3. I'll give you some great recipes for shakes later on in Part Three.

Know the foods that contain omega 3s. The best sources are cold-water fish such as salmon and tuna (or fish oil capsules), flax seeds and flax oil, hemp seeds and hemp oil, and dark green veggies like spinach, kale, seaweed, Japanese greens, and broccoli. You should aim to have at least one serving of these foods per day.

Eat your soy in foods rather than having it as oil

(vegetable oil is soybean oil). Soybeans (which are used to make tofu, soy sauce, and veggie meats, for example) are rich in both omega 6 and omega 3. They also contain fiber, protein, and water, rounding out their nutrition. Although soybeans do contain a high ratio of omega 6 to omega 3, when eaten in foods rather than in oils, the omega 6 isn't as concentrated, plus you get the benefits of the protein, fiber, and flavenoids contained within the foods as well. When the soybeans are made into oil and sold as vegetable oil, the high ratio of omega 6 to omega 3 can really upset your fat balance, especially if you are cooking with lots of it and having it often. So, long story short, avoid vegetable oil, and have your soy as non-GMO tofu, textured vegetable protein, edamame, and miso instead.

Use olive oil for salad dressings, dips, and spreads, and to add flavor to cooked vegetables. Olive oil is better used at room temperature than heated up.

Don't be afraid of avocados. Yes, they have more fat than other veggies (or are they fruits?) but it's healthy, monounsaturated fat. Try a few slices of avocado on a salad or a tablespoon of fresh and creamy guacamole instead of yucky mayo on sandwiches.

Finally, reduce the amount of processed, packaged, and convenient foods you eat; the omega 6 from these adds up quickly.

FAT: THE ULTIMATE FRENEMY •••••••••••••••

As you can see, we need to eat fat, but we need to be mindful of the type and quantity we're eating. We also need to understand that while a little fat is good for nutrition and can help with weight loss, the calories add up quickly. No matter what the source of fat, it all contains

9 calories per gram. That's a lot. It's more than any other food we ingest.

> Here's the calorie tally:
> Fat = 9 calories per gram
> Alcohol = 7 calories per gram
> Protein = 4 calories per gram
> Carbs = 4 calories per gram
> Non-digestible carbs such as certain fibers, sugar alcohols, and fructo-oligosaccharides = 0 calories per gram
> Water = 0 calories per gram
> Air = 0 calories per gram

Naturally, the more fat a product contains, the more caloric it's going to be. A tablespoon of oil contains 14 grams (0.5 ounces) of fat, and at 9 calories per gram, that adds up to a whopping 126 calories. So although olive oil is healthy, if you pour it on top of your veggies and salads without watching the portions, the calories will add up and so will the pounds despite your healthy intentions. Top healthy veggies with 5 tablespoons of oil and you may as well have just had a Big Mac as far as your waistline is concerned. I will give you a good idea of how much is the right amount to be consuming in the meal plans in Part Three.

Bottom line: Eat fat, but be conscious of the types you're eating and how much.

Here are some of my favorite tips for saving on fat calories so that you can afford to indulge in your favorite high-fat foods once in a while. Smart rebels know how to compromise!

Use canned pumpkin instead of butter and eggs in baking. Canned pumpkin actually tastes great mixed with low-fat brownie mixes such as No Pudge! Original Fat Free Fudge Brownie Mix or Bob's Red Mill Brownie Mix. Just stir the pumpkin into the brownie mix and bake. The brownies end up really moist and mousse-like.

Use tasty salad ingredients so that you don't need as much dressing. Good options are freeze-dried fruit, veggie-based bacon bits, like Frontier Certified Organic Bac'uns, fresh fruit, and flavorful veggies such as bell peppers, red onion, jicama, and hearts of palm. Or dilute fattening dressings with vinegar, water, or calorie-free dressings so you can get away with using less of the bad stuff.

Use low-calorie, flavor-packed ingredients when making salad dressings—like flavored vinegars, salt, pepper, garlic, fresh berries, and organic calorie-free sweeteners—so that you need less oil. Or buy ready-made dressings that have already done this for you. See the salad dressing suggestions in Part Two; most of the ones I've selected have fewer than 50 calories in 2 tablespoons, which is pretty darn low considering 2 tablespoons of oil and vinegar rings in at 200 calories.

Try Laughing Cow cheese products, such as their light cheese wedges, and Mini Babybel Light Cheese. These are great!

Bake, barbecue, steam, and boil your foods so that you avoid frying or sautéing in unhealthy oils. Use Spectrum cooking sprays, which use high-quality expeller-pressed oils, instead of butter or oil if you do sauté vegetables and meats; it will cut down on the amount of butter or oil you need, if you need any at all. Plus, it has zero calories and comes in a multitude of varieties. I love the high-heat butter-flavor canola oil spray.

Use Becel Topping and Cooking Spray on potatoes, breads, and vegetables instead of butter or oil. The idea of spraying on this "fake butter," as I've heard it called, grosses some people out, but it shouldn't. It contains no trans fat and no saturated fat, and the first ingredient is water. It does contain soybean oil, but in trace amounts. It's mostly water so it's actually much less gross than clogging your arteries with real margarine (trans fat crap), or heaps of butter (too many calories). Sure, butter's natural, but in my opinion the calories aren't worth it when there's a good alternative available. But when you're having company over, you probably shouldn't spray their food. It's just not classy, even if it is healthier!

Try forgoing dressings, sauces, and butter and see if you notice the change. Many people add butter to foods just out of habit, when really the food tastes pretty darn good without it. Corn on the cob is delicious on its own and doesn't need to be doused with butter. Same for lobster, shrimp, popcorn, and fresh breads. Break the habit; lose the weight.

So fat is an important topic to understand, especially if you want to avoid more of it turning up on your rear end. In case your attention span wavered, here's the synopsis: choose your fat wisely. You can have cream in your coffee, egg yolks in your omelets, cheese on your salads, butter on your toast, and filet mignon at dinner time…but you can't have all of it all of the time or you'll pay the price. You have to compromise and pick your indulgences using lean varieties, substitutes, and smaller portion sizes whenever you can. When you eat something fatty, have a small portion and fill up with lots of high-water, low-calorie foods like fruits, vegetables, and lean meats and fish. This will reduce the fat density for the whole meal. For instance, if you've having steak, skip the baked potato and have a side of steamed vegetables instead. If you're in the mood for pizza, have one slice plus a salad dressed with just balsamic vinegar to fill you up. Up your omega 3 and mono-unsaturated fat intake and drop your saturated fat and trans fat intake, and you'll be well on your way to a hot, healthy bod in no time.

RULE 6:

NO LARGE PORTIONS

(Not gonna happen!)

This rule's just gotta go. We are not little birdies, nor have we had gastric bypasses. We have big tummies, big appetites, and big eyes, and we deserve to feel satisfied and stuffed, even when eating to lose weight.

The biggest mistake I see people make over and over when they are trying to lose weight is not eating enough. It drives me crazy because I know they're trying so hard. I also know that they're setting themselves up for inevitable failure by restricting themselves too much. I see it done in many different ways: there are those who starve themselves all day and then end up binging uncontrollably at night; those who try to restrict themselves to 800 or so calories per day; and those who limit themselves to just a few "safe" foods and eat the same thing every day. Lastly, there are those who think they are blowing their diet by having a large portion of food—even when it's full of low-cal foods like veggies and lean meats. But the thing is, restrictive methods don't work for diets, and they sure as hell don't work for the long term.

I can't tell you how many people I've met who have been on these kinds of restrictive weight loss plans. They usually quit within the first few weeks, or if they stay and endure the torture, they last for a while, lose a lot of weight, and then gain it right back and more as soon as they start eating "normally" again. Nothing was learned. No new lifestyle was adopted. The eating patterns that got them into trouble in the first place are the eating patterns they revert to as soon as they're off the "I'd rather be dead than be on this diet one day longer" plan.

So I find this section incredibly important if you are looking to achieve lasting results. A healthy weight loss plan *can* be endurable, and can even be enjoyable.

BIG PORTIONS, BIG PROBLEMS • • • • • • • • • • • • • •

Before I show you how you can eat like a pig without developing porcine proportions, let's first discuss why big portions have traditionally been discouraged.

Large Portions Have Too Many Calories

In case you still aren't aware of the calorie–weight connection, let me sum if up for you: if you eat more calories than your body requires to function, you will gain weight. Some people need a lot of calories to function, such as athletes and people with inefficient metabolisms or mitochondria (lots of brown fat). They may be able to eat any type of big meal they like without gaining weight…but they're probably not the ones reading this book. You are. You with your normal metabolism and desk job, or you with your thyroid condition and exercise-limiting arthritic knees. And you're reading it because you've eaten one too many big meals one too many times, and now have some impressive hips or chins or rolls to show for it.

The problem with big meals is not their size or bulk or bigness, but rather their tendency to contain loads of calories from fat, protein, and carbs. Take a Big Mac and fries, for example. Actually, please don't take one; just check this out: it has lots of meat, lots of bun and potato, and probably lots of lard, hydrogenated oil, and mayo— protein, carbs, and fat, respectively. That's a lot of calories. And most people don't even fill up on it; instead, they opt to supersize it and maybe add a dessert or soft drink to top it all off. For the price of filling up on this big meal, you can bet your bottom dollar that you're going to have some serious fattening calories to contend with.

The Glycemic Load Is Too High

By now, most of us have heard of the glycemic index. Just to review, though, the glycemic index (GI) is a scale that rates foods by their tendency to raise blood sugar levels. Foods with the highest GI spike blood sugar the most, while those with the lowest GI scores barely raise blood sugar at all. A food's GI is determined by its make-up: the amount of protein, carbs, fat, fiber, and water it contains. But a food's glycemic load is determined by its GI *and* the amount you eat—and that's what matters.

Brown rice has a low GI, but if you eat a couple cups of it, you'll end up with a high glycemic load because you ate so much. White bread has a high GI, but if you eat only one small slice, you'll end up with a fairly low glycemic load because the amount you ate was small. And so it follows that big meals tend to have high glycemic loads because the quantity consumed is high, especially if you eat foods that already have inherently high GI values.

So what do you do if you're forbidden to eat big meals? You either ignore your hunger pangs, opt for stomach-shrinking surgeries like lap bands and gastric bypass procedures, or, most likely, do what most of us do: ignore the rule, eat the big meal, and then deal with being fat and promise yourself you'll go on another diet "tomorrow."

The average adult stomach requires about 2 to 3 pounds of food each day to feel full. (And if you have a history of overeating, you've trained your stomach to want even more.) So unless you fill it up with food or shrink it by surgery, you're going to feel hungry and have cravings. It's our human nature to seek food when we're hungry. That's how we're built, and from an evolutionary perspective it serves us well. But if we shouldn't eat big meals, how can we meet this 3 pound quota? It's simple: by eating big meals. But they have to be calorie-poor, nutrient-rich meals that don't spike blood sugar levels. That's the trick.

In non-geek speak now, you basically have to choose foods that take up lots of space on your plate and in your belly, and therefore take lots of time to eat, but do so for the fewest number of calories. You need to fill up on nutritious foods that are lowest on the calorie ladder. We learned in the last chapter that fat has 9 calories per gram, alcohol has 7 calories per gram, carbs and protein have 4 calories per gram, and fiber, non-digestible carbs, water, and air have absolutely no calories per gram.

Even though protein is stated as having 4 calories per gram, it actually has fewer. This is because our bodies must burn off 30 percent of the calories just to digest and metabolize it. Therefore, what started off as 4 calories becomes

only 2.8 calories by the time this work has
been done. **So protein really has 2.8 calories
per gram, rather than 4 calories.** How cool is
that? Foods that are mostly protein and water, such as chicken breast, turkey breast, egg
whites, game meat, bison, white fish, seafood,
and very lean cuts of red meat, are therefore
superstars for weight loss. As if that wasn't
good enough, because it takes so much time
for our bodies to do this work of digesting,
absorbing, and metabolizing, the food stays
in our stomach for a long time, keeping us full.
Once absorbed into your blood stream, it then
takes even longer for protein to finally be converted to sugar. This means that protein has a
super-low glycemic index, and we stay full and
satisfied for a long time.

When putting together your meals, you want to fill
up on the lower rungs of the ladder—the foods highest in water, air, fiber, and protein—to lower the overall
caloric density of the meal. Instead of having three slices
of pizza with a small salad covered in oil, have one large
slice of thin-crust pizza loaded with veggies with a large
salad full of fibrous vegetables and vinegar-based dressing. The grams of food will be about the same, but the
amount of calories in the second meal will be way, way
less. This takes working at, but it's so worth it because it's
the secret to longevity and a lifetime of leanness.

LIVING LARGE •

Let's look at a whole day of eating to see how this plays
out in real life. I'll compare a day of eating small meals
with a day of eating big meals. The calories consumed
for the day will be the same, but you decide which would
be more satisfying.

Breakfast

Small meal: 2 slices white toast with 2 tablespoons jam

Big meal: 3-egg-white omelet with vegetables and
1 tablespoon shredded light cheddar cheese, 3 slices
Piller's Better than Bacon chicken or turkey bacon, with
1 slice Weight Watchers 100% Whole Wheat Sliced
Bread, toasted and topped with fat-free cream cheese
and sliced tomato

Lunch

Small meal: 1 bagel with tuna salad made with full-fat
mayo

Big meal: 1 miso soup, 1 large La Tortilla Factory
Multi Grain Wrap with vegetables, mustard, and 100
grams (3.5 ounces) of low-fat turkey, 1 single serving of
yogurt, and an apple

Dinner

Small meal: 1 slice of pizza

Big meal: 1 barbecued chicken breast, ½ cup basmati
rice, steamed zucchini, and a side salad with shredded
parmesan and balsamic vinaigrette

Although the small meals weigh less in your stomach
and feel virtuous, I can practically guarantee that from
a weight-loss standpoint, you'd be way better off going
with the big meals. Technically speaking, both days add

up to about the same number of calories, but it would
be harder to resist snacking between meals and having
"seconds" on the small meal day because you'd be so
much hungrier due to the relative lack of fiber, protein,
and volume.

When it comes to big meals, here's what you do:

- Include high-water, low-cal foods like vegetables,
  salads, clear soups, shirataki noodles, berries, grape-
  fruits, and egg whites whenever you can.
- Eat low GI foods such as those listed in the previous
  point, as well as lean meats, fish, and unsweetened
  dairy products, so that you can have more of them
  without spiking sugar levels.
- Limit dry carbs, such as crackers, chips, pretzels,
  cereals, and granola, because the calories add up far
  too quickly. Instead, opt for starches with more water,
  such as whole grain rice, noodles, porridge, and sweet
  potatoes or yams.
- Add flavor with spices, fresh herbs, vinegars, and
  lemon, lime, and orange juice and rind, rather than
  fatty, sugary, oily sauces and dressings—the calories
  add up so quickly that your meal is practically over in
  one or two bites.

Ta da! Now you know how to be naughty licking
your plate clean, ordering seconds, and supersizing your
portions without feeling like you're supersizing your ass
along the way. You should now understand that so long
as you indulge in large amounts of foods that rank low
on the calorie ladder, and modest amounts of those that
rank higher up, you can eat until you're nice and stuffed
without worrying that you're going to morph into King

Kong Bundy overnight. There's nothing sexier than a smart, rebellious chick whose appetite is as healthy as her bodacious bod.

NO BOOZE

(Ha ha!)

Now this is a good rule—if you can follow it. Which, incidentally, I can't.

Booze is bad for diets. It's calorie-rich and nutrient-poor; the opposite of what we want. Alcohol contains 7 calories per gram, almost as much as fat itself. Worse yet, we often mix it with sugary, fatty mixes like cream, soft drinks, and syrups, which further worsens its ranking on the calorie ladder. Add to that the fact that it has virtually no nutrients (just because the OJ you're mixing with your vodka has a little bit of vitamin C doesn't actually make your drink nutritious!), and it's not surprising that most diet books forbid it. And the problems with booze don't end there.

As we all know, alcohol impairs our judgment and lowers our inhibitions. That guy we would normally never have gone home with…oops, never mind that…I mean those chili cheese fries that we normally would never have eaten now seem like a darn good idea. And that bacon, egg, and homefry meal the next morning is practically irresistible.

Alcohol is hard on our livers—duh. So our livers process it immediately after we drink it. Our bodies don't worry about dealing with the fat we've just eaten; they just store that for later (right on top of our tummy rolls, naturally). Instead, our bodies want to get rid of the alcohol. Personally, I'd prefer my body work on the fat while I enjoy my buzz guilt-free, but it doesn't work like that.

As you can see, alcohol is not the best idea for weight loss. That being said, if you enjoy the odd drink—which I'm sure many a rebel does—it's not an automatic deal breaker. At the risk of sounding redundant, the dose makes the poison, people. So a glass of wine with dinner, or a few too many on a special occasion, or heck, even a margarita by the pool won't ruin your hard work if you keep it limited and imbibe wisely.

BEATING THE BEER GUT

First of all, watch how much you're drinking. From a health standpoint, it's recommended that women aim to have two or fewer drinks per day, and men aim for three or fewer per day. From a calorie standpoint, the less you consume the better, since the calories add up quickly. One bar shot (44 milliliters or 1.5 ounces) of a clear alcoholic spirit, such as vodka, whiskey, gin, rum, or tequila, has about 90 calories. One 150 milliliter (5 ounce) glass of wine has about 100 calories, and one 341 milliliter (12 ounce) bottle of beer has about 150 calories. (That's a whopping 900 calories if you drink a six-pack a day.) Light beer is a tiny bit better at 100 calories per bottle.

Choose your mixes wisely. Although a shot of rum may have only 90 calories, if you're mixing it with 175 milliliters (6 ounces) of cola each time, you'll end up drinking 160 calories. And of course it will go down way too quickly because of the sweet taste. You're better off sticking to calorie-free, sugar-free mixes such as water, soda water, or—last resort—diet soft drinks. It may not taste as good, but it will have fewer calories and less sugar, and it will take longer to drink.

Despite the "watery" name, tonic water is not a good choice. It's not calorie-free like plain water or soda water. In fact, tonic water packs a whopping 90 calories in a cup. Mix your gin or vodka with soda water and squeezed lime wedges instead of tonic. If you find the taste of vodka and soda too bland, try one of the new flavor-infused vodkas, like citrus or vanilla vodka. They only have 5 more calories per ounce than regular vodka (69 calories, compared to 64), but they have quite a bit of flavor.

Also, be careful with cutesy-sounding, girly-looking martinis. They often contain two shots of booze in addition to the mix, and will end up having from 230 calories per martini (in a cosmo, for instance) to over 400 calories. (A chocolate martini has 430 calories—more than a Snickers bar!) Plus, they're so tiny and yummy that they'll go down quickly, the calories will add up, and next thing you know you'll be drinking too fast for your liver…and your waistline, not to mention your judgment and your barf threshold. If you must have a martini, sip on a seemingly unappealing one instead, like a dirty martini. Made with gin, vermouth, and olive brine, it rings in at about 200 calories, and you'll probably sip it slowly—it's pretty hard to chug back olive brine.

At the beach, don't sacrifice your hard-earned bikini body! Avoid those deadly blender drinks. One 175 milliliter (6 ounce) pina colada has 630 calories. So you'd better really love it, or it just ain't worth it, hon. A similar-sized strawberry margarita has slightly fewer calories (about 450), but still, is it worth it? You decide. If you need to cool off, jump in the water and swim some calories off instead.

Don't be fooled by so-called low carb beer, thinking it means "indulge without guilt." It doesn't. Low carb beer is

not really low in carbs; it's just *lower* in carbs than regular
beer. It's also typically lower in alcohol. But it's not really
"low carb." After all, all alcohol contains carbs. What do
you think it's made from? Grain, potatoes, and grapes—all
carbs. The carbohydrate is fermented to make alcohol,
so alcohol is just fermented (i.e., rotten—yucky!) carbs.
In fact, alcohol is a concentrated form of carb that has 7
calories per gram instead of the usual 4 calories per gram
that your non-rotten carbs have. And it raises blood sugar
and spikes insulin just like standard carbs.

When beer is marketed as low carb, what it means is
that more of the carb (the barley, for instance) is fermented into alcohol. Because it has a higher alcohol percentage, it's then diluted with water to give you an end
product that is similar in alcohol content to regular beer
but with slightly fewer carbs and calories. For example,
Bud Light has 110 calories, 4.2 percent alcohol, and 6.6
grams (0.2 ounces) of carbs per 341 milliliter (12 ounce)
bottle, and a bottle of good old regular Bud has 145 calories, 5.0 percent alcohol, and 10.6 grams (0.4 ounces) of
carbs. In essence, you save yourself 35 calories and get
a little less carb when you go with a Bud Light, but you
also get less alcohol. If you're planning on chugging back
a six-pack, this will make a difference; if you're just having one, the savings aren't really worth much. And really,
you could just make low carb beer yourself by pouring
out a little beer from a regular bottle and filling it back
up with water.

Wine can be a good option because it doesn't come
contaminated with any gross mixes. (Unless you make
the mistake of ordering a wine cooler. Don't—the wine is
mixed with fruit juice, sugar, and a carbonated beverage,

so it packs heaps of sugar and calories.) Plus, you can sip a glass of wine slowly, so it can last a while. That being said, it's also easy to pack on pounds quickly if you start drinking wine on a daily basis with dinner. Since classy rebels associate wine with romance, relaxation, sophistication, and even health, it's easy to fall into the trap of allowing yourself to split a bottle with your hubby every evening. Even if you skipped high school math, it doesn't take a genius to bust out a calculator and figure out that if you have two or three glasses of wine (half a bottle) a day, at 100 calories per glass you'll end up ingesting about 1,750 calories for the week just from wine. Which will result in you packing on a pound of fat every two weeks, since 3,500 calories results in a pound of fat. Or think about it this way instead: if you do nothing else but cut out the habit, you'll save yourself 1,750 calories per week and lose a half a pound of fat every week without changing your eating habits at all.

Booze doesn't have to be all bad, and can even work to your benefit in a way. Because alcohol contains calories (in other words, energy) and removes your usual good judgment, it's the perfect excuse to get moving and dance, regardless of how funny your less-than-stellar moves may look. You might as well burn off some of those empty calories!

Of course, if alcohol is problematic for you and you can't enjoy a drink or two without eating the entire contents of your fridge, rebel against the cocktail crowd and avoid it altogether. It's not worth ruining your hard work for. You won't even remember eating all that food anyway. (Which doesn't mean it won't count—sadly, calories still count even if you've blocked the memory out.) If you don't want to hang at home while your friends hit the club, opt for these fakey drinks instead and no one will know the difference:

- Soda water mixed with a little cranberry juice and a wedge of lemon
- Diet cola with a wedge of lime
- Virgin Bloody Mary or Virgin Bloody Caesar
- An energy drink (preferably a diet one, if they have it) with a wedge of lemon on the side

HANGOVER HELL •

Since alcohol is a major diuretic, it causes our balance of water and electrolytes to get all out of whack. As a result, our bodies feel sluggish and weak, our brains feel fuzzy, and our bellies crave foods concentrated in sugar and salt to try to rebalance our body chemistry. The key to avoiding hangover hell (other than moderation, of course!) is to drink a glass of water for every alcoholic drink you consume, and to down some extra water before bed to minimize dehydration. If you don't manage to dodge that bullet, you're doomed to crave salty, greasy, diet-destroying foods. Eating salt and sugar causes us to retain water, which is what our body wants to do to rehydrate. Rather than reaching for the chips, bacon, fries, and processed, high-salt foods, though, reach for salty soups, beverages, and foods that are less damaging

to your waistline, and at least pack in some good nutrition and water content as well. Have a Greek salad with
salty feta cheese and a V8. Or have a veggie burger with
pickles and tomato soup. You catch my drift—get the salt
and sugar your body craves, but do it intelligently.

Hangovers also stem from alcohol and sugar withdrawal. When our body withdraws from large amounts
of both, we feel the effects on our sympathetic nervous
system: fast heart rate, shaky hands, pounding heads,
and nausea. The last thing you want to do when in this
state is further speed up the system by drinking caffeine-
packed coffee or energy drinks. They'll make you feel
worse and more dehydrated. You can minimize these annoying aftereffects by avoiding sugary mixes so you have
less sugar to withdraw from.

Lastly, hangover hell stems from an accumulation of
toxins. After all, your liver was busy processing the booze,
so it wasn't able to work on detoxifying and eliminating
the other toxins you encountered. Don't add to this toxic
load the next day by adding processed foods and soft
drinks full of chemicals to the mix. Have a healthy day—
do a little exercise, drink water, and eat clean.

So now that we've tackled alcohol—the good, the bad,
and the ugly—I encourage you to consider my tips the
next time you raise a glass. But also take a good, hard look
at your drinking patterns and really gauge whether alcohol is a problem for you. Is it affecting your health goals?
Your weight loss goals? Your relationships? Your work?
Your family? If the answer to any of the above is yes,
please talk to your doctor about some ways to seek help.

NO COFFEE

(I don't think so!)

For years now, we've been hearing how coffee can be detrimental to our diet, while tea—especially green tea—is extremely beneficial for both our health and our waistlines. There's no disputing the latter: green tea is certainly healthy and a rich source of antioxidants and calorie-burning catechins (more on this in a bit). But coffee, as we're learning, isn't so bad either.

Get this: coffee is the number one source of antioxidants in the North American diet. It's also fat-free, virtually calorie-free, metabolism-boosting, and appetite-suppressing. So why on earth is coffee banned in almost all diet programs? I think the reason for this rule—which we're totally going to break; not to worry—is multifold: it dehydrates us, distracts us, stimulates us, and tricks us. Here's how.

DEHYDRATION

Coffee is a diuretic. It causes us to pee a lot, and when we pee, we flush water as well as important electrolytes such as sodium, potassium, magnesium, and calcium directly from our bodies down the toilet. So basically, instead of nourishing and hydrating us, which is what we want from our diet, it does the exact opposite. Fine. But really, is it that bad? I mean, for us rebels, isn't a little flush okay, especially if toxins get flushed out as well?

Yes, but…to avoid losing nutrients and dehydrating, it's important to limit coffee consumption to no more than two or three cups per day. And, it's very important to drink water throughout the day and to ensure that you are eating a balanced diet. Taking a daily multivitamin is also a good idea, for insurance. Our bodies often confuse the sensations of hunger and thirst, so if you dehydrate from a morning's worth of coffee, you may experience major afternoon hunger pangs and fatigue due to thirst. In other words, your body is thirsty for water, yet you interpret the sensation as hunger and exhaustion and wolf down a muffin, with, gasp, another coffee—and this is the problem.

Drinking coffee is okay, but you do not want to get into the cycle of dehydration and hunger. That will set you up for failure, so a good rule of thumb is to match every cup of coffee you drink with a glass of water. Also, when hunger rolls around in the afternoon, try drinking some water first and then reassessing the situation in 15 minutes. It may just do the trick to satisfy your hunger.

DISTRACTION •

Coffee is tasty, warm, and comforting. Great! But it's been bashed on many a diet plan for exactly these reasons. It distracts us from experimenting with other tasty, warm, and comforting beverages—tea, in particular. Let's look at tea.

Tea can be white, green, oolong (red), and black. All tea, regardless of the color, derives its leaves from the tree known as *Camellia sinensis*. These tea leaves are extremely high in antioxidant polyphenols, which is why tea gets such a good rap. It's so beneficial for our health and has been implicated in lowering our risk for heart disease, stroke, and various cancers. It also helps strengthen our immune system and promotes longevity, and can even help us lose weight.

What about the colors? The color of the tea reflects how much it's been processed and therefore what type of polyphenol it contains. The lighter teas—white and green—are the least processed and contain the most catechin polyphenols. These catechins boost metabolism and curb appetite, and that is why white and green tea have been shown to help people lose weight. They're calorie burners, so you should drink a cup after meals for maximum effect—which will also help you from going back to the fridge for seconds. Oolong and black tea are more processed and therefore darker in color. They contain loads of polyphenols, so they're still excellent for our health, but they contain less of the metabolism-boosting catechins, which is why they're not mentioned as much in diet books. Also, unlike green tea, which people tend to drink straight up, black tea is often topped up with milk and sugar, which reduces its health benefits.

Beyond the added calories, the protein in milk, casein, can bind to the polyphenols, preventing them from working. So if you want to reap the benefits of black tea, you'll have to get used to drinking it black. Squeeze a lemon into it, or if you must have a milky taste, add unsweetened almond milk or soy milk, which do not contain casein.

Before we get back to coffee, I want to mention one final thing about herbal tea and rooibos tea. These so-called teas aren't really teas at all; they are simply infusions made from herbs, roots, flowers and spices. They aren't made from *Camellia sinensis* leaves, so they don't pack the polyphenol benefits. But they're yummy, calorie-free, and caffeine-free, so they have a lot of pros on their own. Personally, I love licorice spice herbal "tea;" it tastes sweet and is great to sip after dinner so you don't attack the cookie cupboard instead.

STIMULATION ••••••••••••••••••••••••••••

Coffee—well, the caffeine in it actually—is an adenosine receptor antagonist. Um, come again? When I worked for a summer in Winnipeg as a lab tech/research assistant, one of the students working alongside me actually had that sentence taped to his giant coffee mug. (Incidentally, he also helped me guillotine rats for the advancement of science. I didn't last long at that job.) Anyhow...

Caffeine blocks adenosine, which is a calming neurotransmitter, so it stimulates us, wakes us up, and exacerbates nervousness, tension, and anxiety in the process. This can be a good thing or a bad thing for weight loss, depending on what you do in this aroused state. If you take advantage of the high and exercise, it's a great thing. Studies have shown that drinking coffee before a workout can actually increase strength and stamina and help you train longer and harder. But if you're the type that nervously munches, nibbles, and picks when you're buzzing, it's a bad thing. My advice, then, is to avoid becoming overly stimulated, by limiting coffee to an amount that wakes you to an alert calm rather than a hyper buzz, and by following up your cup with either physical or mental work.

TRICKERY ••••••••••••••••••••••••••••••

It poses as sugar-free, fat-free, and calorie-free, but if we're not astute, this coy cup of "coffee" can be anything

but. I mean, have you seen the calories in a Starbucks
Frappuccino or a Tim Hortons Iced Capp? Have you
seen the treats and sweets that people indulge in on their
"coffee break," or the amounts of cream and sugar that
people add mindlessly to their java? My friend, when
you drink it like that, coffee is a diabolical diet disaster.

Everyday coffee, the bitter-tasting black beverage
made from coffee beans, is fat-free, sugar-free, and
almost calorie-free. But "coffee," the frothy, sprinkled, icy
thing with a seven-word name, topped with oil-based
whipped cream and alongside a stale pastry, is not.

If you're going to indulge in coffee while trying to
lose weight, you need to take an honest look at how
you take it and whether that is standing in the way of
your success. If you add cream and sugar, you may be
okay—if you stick to just a cup. If you have cup after cup,
however, you will need to make some changes because
the calories will add up quickly. If you can't go out for
a coffee break without picking up something sweet or
crunchy or chewy along with it, then you'll have to stop
breaking for coffee; it's just that simple.

My first tip for having your coffee and drinking it too
is to drink no more than two or three cups per day max.
But also avoid the temptation to eat something with your
coffee. This is a habit that you can easily break with a
little practice. Look forward to the coffee itself. Try new
flavors and new brands, and really savor each sip. I have
a friend who wakes up each morning looking forward to
her "juicy" coffee (it's not juicy at all, obviously, but she
thinks of it this way). She drinks it slowly, savoring the
aroma and taste of each sip. If drinking coffee is really
about the snacks or sweets that go along with it, then
skip it.

Avoid fancy coffee concoctions served at restaurants
and cafes. Although they sound harmless enough, they
tend to have loads of calories, fat, and sugar. Even skinny
or light varieties can be loaded with calories (just check
out the nutritional information on the Starbucks website
for a jolt of a different sort). If you want an iced coffee
treat, blend a cup of unsweetened almond milk with
crushed ice, a teaspoon of instant coffee, some vanilla
extract, and a teaspoon of organic coffee creamer (or
Coffee-mate Lite). It's just as good as an iced cappuccino,
but way better for you.

Try to wean yourself off sugar in your coffee. I did,
and I like it tons more now. If you must have it sweet, try
my natural sweetener suggestions on page 132.

Watch out for flavored syrups. The full-calorie ones
pack loads of calories—just a three-pump dose of flavored syrup has 60 calories and 15 grams (about half an
ounce) of sugar. To save yourself the sugar grams, you
can opt for the calorie-free syrups, but bear in mind that
they can induce serious gas and diarrhea from the heaps
of sugar alcohols used. Just avoid these all together and
try flavoring your coffee with cinnamon or almond milk.
Personally, I add cinnamon to my coffee grounds before
brewing a pot, and it tastes delicious! If you must indulge
in flavor shots, just ask your barista to use one shot
instead of the usual three.

Watch out for the milk. Although milk, especially
skim, has fewer calories than cream, if you add half a cup
into each coffee, or consume latte after latte, the calories
will quickly add up. For example, two medium (grande)
skinny lattes without whipped cream or flavored syrups will still tally up to a whopping 260 calories and

36 grams (1.3 ounces) of sugar. Holy crap! If you have a medium, non–skim milk latte with—gasp—a flavor, such as a pumpkin spice latte, you'll take in almost 400 calories just for one. That innocent-sounding "vegetable" latte doesn't sound so innocent anymore, does it? Heck, you'd be better off having a soft drink. And don't think that a tea latte is any better—a grande Tazo Chai Tea Latte at Starbucks rings in at 240 calories and 41 grams (1.5 ounces) of sugar. Hmm…do you think it's the caffeine that's making your Starbucks run addictive, or all the sugar that comes along with it? To avoid packing on the pounds drinking coffee, you're better off having a cup or two of coffee with a tablespoon or so of cream in each—that will only set you back 30 calories. Or just try it black to keep it totally fat-free. After all, they say that once you go black, you never go back!

If you use these tips, you can enjoy coffee without derailing your diet in the process. In fact, the latest research shows that not only is coffee safe, but it can actually help you lose weight.

Coffee speeds up metabolism, which means you burn a few extra calories while at rest. It also gives you energy for a longer, more intense workout, which will burn calories in the process and keep your metabolism revved for hours after. Although people once believed that coffee consumption increased the risk for heart disease and diabetes, the latest research doesn't support this. Studies show that four to five cups a day can actually reduce the risk of Type 2 diabetes by as much as 30 percent. And the Health Professionals Follow-up Study, which followed 45,000 men for several years, found that total coffee intake was not associated with coronary heart disease or stroke, even when men drank more than four cups per day.

What about the toxins or potential carcinogens in coffee beans? You may have heard about this, but if you haven't, sorry to freak you out. It's been reported that coffee contains nearly twenty chemicals deemed possible carcinogens in animals. But coffee hasn't triggered cancer in animals, and there is no reported study linking coffee and cancer. Weird? Not really. Remember, the dose makes the poison, so even though these toxins are present, the concentration is too low to do any harm. In fact, it's just the opposite. Coffee is a rich source of anti-cancer polyphenols, and, as I mentioned earlier, is actually the richest source of antioxidants in the North American diet—partially because it's a good source, but also because we drink so much of the stuff. The bottom line: if you like coffee, you can have it, but follow the tips I've given you to ensure that you're not jeopardizing your health and weight-loss goals. And if you don't like coffee, or if it keeps you up at night, or if you'd prefer tea, then don't worry either. You don't have to drink coffee; I'm just saying that on my plan, you can.

NO QUITTING

(Unlikely!)

This sounds like a good rule. After all, no one likes a quitter. But when we're talking about dieting down to unrealistic weights, we need to quit it. We're all made to be different shapes, sizes, and proportions—unique snowflakes of human beings—so it's ridiculous to think we all need to be a size zero to be healthy. So how do you know how much you should aim to weigh?

THE MEASURING TAPE

A good rule of thumb is to aim for an abdominal circumference of less than 35 inches for women and 40 inches for men. Above this and you can bet your booty than you're storing excess, inflammatory visceral fat.

THE SCALE

This is a weighty issue. No one likes the scale, but it really is the best way to tell how your weight-loss plan is progressing. Think of it metaphorically as a bank account: if you don't check the balance, how do you know if your savings plan is working? That being said, do *not* obsessively check the scale. Instead, weigh yourself just once weekly and aim for a healthy 2 pound loss per week. If you have a lot to lose, you may lose more than 2 pounds a week, and if you have less to lose, the amount per week may be slightly lower. Also, be aware that even if you do everything "right," the scale may not always reflect your efforts in the same way each week. Don't self-sabotage if this happens by bingeing on everything in sight; this is the worst mistake you can make. Some weeks you may be disgruntled or downright pissed off that you've only lost a quarter of a pound, and some weeks you may be amazed to see that you've suddenly dropped 4 pounds. As long as the weight is trending down over time, you're on track.

As you lose weight, you should expect to encounter plateaus periodically. Your body is just re-adjusting. Weight loss tends to be more rapid at the beginning of the plan because as you deplete your glycogen stores, you lose water weight as well as fat. Once you are on the plan for a while, you experience mostly fat loss, so you won't see as drastic a drop on the scale. But it is even more important that you stick with your plan at this stage, because now you're into the real fat loss. This is the weight that you want to lose: the visceral and subcutaneous fat stores. I see too many people start a diet, lose 10 pounds quickly, plateau for a bit, and then revert right back to their old habits and gain the weight right back. They do this over and over, but really all they're doing is losing water and gaining water; no real fat loss is taking place. You need to stick with the plan, even through plateaus, to see ongoing results. To reach your goal, the Three Ps—patience, persistence, and a positive attitude—are just as integral to success as your new eating habits.

Body Mass Index

When you're thinking of setting a weight loss goal, you should also calculate your Body Mass Index (BMI). To calculate your BMI, multiply your weight in pounds by 703 and then divide this result by your height in inches squared. Here's the formula:

BMI = weight in pounds × 703 ÷ (height in inches × height in inches)

Or just go to the National Institutes of Health website and plug your weight and height into their BMI calculator (www.nhlbisupport.com/bmi).

Your ideal BMI is between 18.5 and 25. Anything above 25 is considered overweight, anything above 30 is considered obese, and anything above 40 is considered morbidly obese. Now, before you curse my name for even suggesting that your BMI of 41 renders you morbidly obese, hear me out.

I don't rely that much on BMI when I set goals with patients. Instead, I look at the shape of their bodies, where the majority of their weight is stored, their blood work, their genetics, their eating habits, their history, and their abdominal circumferences. Sometimes we decide that a BMI below 25 is not realistic and probably not even necessary. Remember that any weight loss is beneficial—you can and will see significant improvements in your health with a reduction of a mere 10 percent of your body weight—so let that be your first goal. In other words, if you weigh 200 pounds, make it your first goal to drop 20 pounds. Think in baby steps and reset your goals often. Visit your doctor before you embark on a weight-loss plan and set goals together.

In addition to setting your BMI, the scale also helps determine the length of the string on your yo-yo. It's normal for your weight to fluctuate: PMS, vacations, holidays, and stressful life events happen to all of us and often result in weight changes. The key is monitoring how much of a change your body registers and knowing when you need to put the brakes on. Again, let's go back to our bank account metaphor. There are times in our life when we have to spend more—birthdays, holidays, etc.—but this doesn't mean we have to go into major debt each time we hit the bank. Same with your weight. I understand that you may gain a few pounds while on vacation or during the holidays, but it's how much you let yourself slip that will determine the length of your yo-yo string. Slight 5-pound variations are normal and acceptable, but 50-pound fluctuations are not. Set a goal weight range and stick to it. The scale will help keep you honest. So will your clothing.

YOUR CLOTHING •

If your clothes are getting tight, you're gaining weight. If your pants are getting shorter despite the fact that you haven't grown an inch since your sixteenth birthday, you're gaining weight. If your shirt buttons are popping open, you're gaining weight. If you've stopped wearing your favorite jeans, the ones you spent a small fortune on, you've gained the weight, hon. Sorry. Don't waste your time blaming the drier or the drycleaner or the fabric; just accept the situation and take the hint. Don't ask your friends or family if you're fat. If your clothes aren't fitting, something got bigger. Probably you. The truth sucks.

THE MIRROR •

Except for porn stars and exhibitionists, no one likes
how they look naked. You can bet your ass that some-
where right this minute there's a supermodel standing
naked in front of her mirror hating the look of her thighs
or hips or fat knees or whatever. My point is, don't obsess
about how you look in the mirror to determine your goal
weight. And please, don't ever let it discourage you or
take away from your weight-loss successes. Instead, love
your body and set a goal to be healthy. Once you reach
your health goal and have healthy eating habits, control
over emotional binges, a healthy weight range, and improvements in your blood sugar and cholesterol, then do
what you gotta do to fake the rest. The best eating habits
in the world won't defeat gravity or an ill-advised outfit.
Love your body, eat for health, lose unhealthy visceral
fat, and then the rest is up to you. And don't fuck it all
up by dressing fat. Seriously, don't. Your goal is a healthy,
strong body. Once you achieve that, dress for success and
blow peoples' socks off with how great you look.

To help, I've got some fab tips to make your new
bod look even better. First of all, wear an overall mono-
chromatic look whenever you can. A black top with
black pants, set off with a colored open blazer, cardigan,
or shawl over top, will look great and keep a long, clean
line. Avoid wearing a top and bottom in radically different colors—peoples' eyes will register where the difference hits and they'll think you're heavier than you are.

Don't even think about trends that don't suit your
body type or age. Just because you've lost 50 pounds and
look amazing doesn't mean you should go out and buy

thigh-high boots, white jeans, or a mini skirt. So what if they're in style? If you're fifty and you're trying to pull off a cheap tube top, the only thing "in" will be you and trouble.

Use vertical lines and stripes to your advantage. They draw the eye up and down so peoples' brains think tall and skinny. Avoid horizontal stripes, especially anywhere near trouble areas. (Doesn't the American flag look kind of fat to you? Kidding!)

Recruit a tailor to make your clothes fit perfectly. If you think something is bulging or pulling, it is. Don't ask your best friend for her opinion. She'll be nice. Your tailor won't. He'll fix it.

Avoid baggy clothing. I understand that you may *feel* thin in them, since they drape off you, but they certainly do nothing to help you *look* thin. Anorexics wear baggy clothing to hide their extreme weight loss; the last thing you, a healthy-weight woman, want to do is hide your hard-earned weight loss. Flaunt how great you look! Wear clothes that hug you in all the right spots.

Explore the world of body shapers. The creations out there these days are truly amazing. You may have heard of Spanx body-shaping undergarments (if not, definitely go to www.spanx.com), but now there's body-shaping apparel that thins and shapes you beautifully as well. Check out www.yummietummie.com.

Let ruching be your new word of the day. Ruching is amazing. Gathered fabric adds curves to less shapely frames and thins out heavier ones. If you're feeling fat or bloated or boyish or whatever, wear a dress or shirt with ruching.

Don't add the look of extra weight to your legs. Avoid patterned hosiery and clunky, heavy shoes. (Unless you're actually in the water, do NOT wear Crocs.) For the appearance of long, lean legs, wear camel-colored or skin-tone high-heeled shoes and avoid ankle straps, opting for slingbacks when you can.

Wear a heel, if you can. High heels really elongate the leg and make you stand up taller. Plus, they give your calves a workout in the process. Nothing disguises a cankle better than a beautiful camel-colored heel.

So there you have it. Set a realistic goal, stick with it, track your progress honestly with the help of your scale and clothing, and then wow everyone with how great you look! Sounds like a plan to me. And speaking of plans, now that you've learned the art of breaking lame, outdated diet rules, let's start putting your specific Rebel Diet weight loss plan into action. In Part Two, we're going to start walking the walk as we grab our imaginary shopping carts and head to the grocery store together. Once you're equipped with the right ingredients, shedding pounds and feeling fantastic is right around the corner. Hallelujah!

PART TWO

THE GOODS— THAT WE'RE GOING TO BUY AND MAKE

Okay ladies, get ready—we're about to go shopping together. My favorite activity in the whole wide world! We're not buying clothing, shoes, or jewelry (frown), but what we are buying is still exciting: groceries! Delicious, healthy groceries that are going to spark your imagination and excite your taste buds while helping you achieve that gorgeous, fit body you deserve.

My clients, friends, and colleagues always ask me to suggest specific products and foods for them, so I've spent the last year researching and testing the latest and greatest products. I can't believe I'm giving away my secrets. I'm having a bit of separation anxiety...but I'll get over it. Let's go shopping!

In this part, we're going to hit the grocery store together. I've sorted food products into categories that closely emulate the layout of your typical grocery store. We'll hit the fresh market first, where you'll pick up your produce, baked goods, dairy, and deli items, and then we'll cruise up and down the aisles, where you'll find frozen foods, beverages, cereals, canned goods, and more. Most of the items can be found at your local supermarket, so that's a good place to start. You can also look for items at specialty grocers like Whole Foods, Trader Joes, and your local health food and organic stores. If you're still having trouble tracking down some of the goodies, order them online via www.amazon.com, www.lowcarbgrocery.com, www.locarbu.com, www.netrition.com, or the product website. And don't be too shy to ask your local grocer to order items in. Finally, rest assured that although I'm a proud Canuck, practically all of the items are found on both sides of the border, but when they're on one side only, I'll let you know.

You'll notice that the list of grocery suggestions is pages and pages long. Don't freak out and think you have to go out and buy all of them at once. You don't! Instead, read through and see what catches your eye. Choose a few new items to try each week or month. Highlight items to look forward to. The plan is to not get bored eating the same thing day in and day out.

In Part Three, I've included suggestions and recipes for how you can use many of the products, so read through Part Three before you go shopping and decide what meals you're going to try each week, then buy what you need. Also check out the product websites, because they're often chock full of tips, tricks, and recipes. Do this especially with foods that are new to you, such as House Foods Tofu Shirataki noodles or Truvia sweetener. On the websites for both products, you'll find lots of fun, tasty, rebel-friendly recipes to try. It's all about experimenting and opening your mind—and your kitchen—to new ideas.

CHAPTER 10

FRESH MARKET

BAKERY •

Breads

There are lots of great bread options on the market now that are delicious and satisfying without breaking the calorie/carb bank. These are some of my favorite items.

For bread products such as crackers, bread, bagels, tortillas, and pitas, I will let you know how much equals one serving (typically it's between 80 and 130 calories). In the meal plans in Part Three, feel free to swap breads as you choose, so long as you stick to the serving size. For instance, you could interchange two slices of Weight Watchers 100% Whole Wheat Sliced Bread or one La Tortilla Factory Multi Grain Wrap or one slice of Dimpflmeier Pumpernickel Bread—they all equal one bread serving.

Food for Life Ezekiel 4:9 Organic Sprouted 100% Whole Grain Flourless Bread: This bread is loaded with protein and fiber, making it an excellent low-glycemic choice. One slice has 80 calories and can be counted as one bread serving.

Food for Life Ezekiel 4:9 Pocket Bread: One pocket has only 100 calories and is considered one bread serving.

Food for Life Genesis 1:29 Organic Sprouted Grain & Seed Bread: This bread is also delicious and high in fiber and protein, and one slice equals one bread serving.

Dimpflmeier Pumpernickel Bread *(Canada*; also available in the US via www.dimpfbreadex.com): One slice equals 80 calories, and the first ingredient is spring water—so healthy! This bread is great. One slice is one bread serving.

Weight Watchers 100% Whole Wheat Sliced Bread: This is a really good product, high in fiber and protein. One slice has only 45 calories, so two slices is equivalent to one bread serving. I love making French Toast with this bread! See page 163 for my recipe.

Nature's Own 100% Whole Wheat Bread: The first two ingredients are stone ground whole wheat and water. Two slices equal one bread serving.

Wonder Light Wheat Bread: Wonder Bread has finally caught on to the health trend! Two slices, packed with protein and fiber, have only 80 calories and equal one bread serving.

Thomas' Original English Muffins: This is a great brand. One muffin counts as one bread serving. If you can find them, Thomas' also has a 100-calorie version that's even lighter. **Wonder Plus**, **Weight Watchers**, and **PC Blue Menu** *(Canada)* also make very good English muffins. English muffins are awesome for making a healthy breakfast sandwich—just cook some egg whites

and add one slice of low-fat cheese and a slice of
Canadian bacon.

**La Tortilla Factory Multi Grain Wraps, Mama Lupe
Tortillas, and Food for Life Whole Grain Brown Rice
Tortillas:** These are all great brands that taste awesome
and are super-low in calories. You can eat a whole tortilla
for one bread serving. Grab them at most health food
stores or online at www.lowcarbgrocery.com and www.
locarbu.com. Have fun using them to make lunch wraps,
fajitas, quesadillas, and pizzas.

Bagels: When I think of Sunday mornings, I think of
bagels, lox, and cream cheese. Yum! But when you're
watching your waistline, bagels are tricky—they often
pack 300 or more calories. **Weight Watchers** makes a
bagel that's pretty waistline-friendly at only 150 calories
(two bread servings). You can also try **Baker's Deluxe
High Fibre Bagels**, but be warned—although they are
amazingly filling and delicious and have only 90 calories (one bread serving), they can cause serious gas and
bloating. (At least they did for me, but not for one of
my clients, so it's worth experimenting. Don't make date
plans for that night, just in case!)

Breadcrumbs: If you're going to use breadcrumbs in
your cooking, do so in moderation and opt for one of
these brands: **Edward and Sons Organic Breadcrumbs**
(the Italian Herbs breadcrumbs are great), **Kikkoman
Panko Bread Crumbs**, or **Ian's Panko Breadcrumbs**.
(Panko breadcrumbs are crispier, airier, and lower in calories than regular breadcrumbs—and they're delicious!)

DELI •••••••••••••••••••••••••••••••••••••

Deli Cheeses and Dips

Dofino Light Havarti Slices: One slice is a great snack melted on a piece of bread or **Ziggy's Internationale Havarti Light Cheese Slices** *(Canada).*

Fresh grated Parmesan cheese: A 2 tablespoon serving has only 40 calories and adds such flavor to omelets, salads, sauces, and cooked veggies.

Hummus: There are lots of great brands to choose from. Hummus is a delicious, super-healthy dip for veggies and adds tons of flavor to sandwiches. A little goes a long way, so try to use no more than 2 tablespoons at a time.

Summer Fresh is my favorite brand; the regular hummus has only 25 calories per tbsp and tastes fantastic and they even have an Edamame Hummus that has 30 calories per tbsp. Check out the Snack'n Go! selections as well. The Hummus & Flatbread Snack'n Go! has only 150 calories and is an excellent mid afternoon snack.

Deli Meats

Tyson Fully Cooked Grilled Chicken Breast or Steak Strips *(US):* These are really great. Just toss them into a salad or sandwich, and you're ready to go.

Lean turkey, chicken, and ham: Deli meats are great to have on hand. Opt for meats that are free of nitrites and low in sodium whenever you can. **Hormel 100 Percent Natural Deli Meats** *(US)* offers some good options, as do **PC Blue Menu** and **Ziggy's** *(Canada).*

Lilydale Fully Cooked Sliced Chicken Breasts
(Canada): These are ready to go, and they taste amazing!
They really come in handy when you're having one of
those days (or lives): you're on the go, super-busy, and
running around like a...on second thought, never mind
that expression.

PC Blue Menu Sliced Chicken Breasts *(Canada)*:
Awesome—fully cooked, ready to eat, and no nitrites. If
they're not in the deli section of your grocery store, try
looking in the refrigerated section, where the hot dogs
and bacon are located.

Maple Leaf Simply Savour Grilled Meat Strips
(Canada): Chicken, turkey, and steak—you just heat
these up in the microwave for 30 seconds and done. It
makes adding protein to your meals easier than ever.
Check out www.greatmealsinminutes.com for cooking
ideas. If you can't find these in the deli section of your
grocery store, try looking in the refrigerated section.

Breakfast Meats

Low-fat strip bacon: Bacon is delicious, but so high in
fat. Try these lower calorie versions instead to save your
waistline: **Wellshire Organic Turkey Bacon** or **Piller's
Tastes Better than Bacon** (hickory smoked turkey,
chicken, or honey maple smoked ham).

Back bacon (aka Canadian bacon): This style of bacon
is prepared from pork loin, so it's actually quite lean—
much leaner than strip bacon. **Schneiders Canadian
Back Bacon** *(Canada)* has only 50 calories for four

slices. Wow! It's already fully cooked, so just heat it up in the microwave or skillet for a great protein-packed addition to your breakfast. Hormel *(US)* also makes a good Canadian bacon.

PRODUCE •
Because fruits and vegetables are so healthy, nutritious, and high in water content, I encourage you to fill up your refrigerator with as many as possible (except for dried fruit and fruit packed in sugary syrups, of course). Here are some of my absolute staples, as well as specific suggestions for awesome fresh fruits and vegetables that you may not be familiar with.

Veggies
Arugula: This leafy green has so much flavor, and it's fantastic in salads. It's also great wilted, so whenever I make something hot, like chicken and vegetables or omelets, I lay a bed of arugula down on my plate first.

Kale: Go ahead, try it; don't be scared. This is literally one of the best foods in the world. It has super-high nutrient density and super-low caloric density—exactly what we want! And it's so easy to use. Just tear it into pieces and steam, or better yet, make kale chips. They're amazing! See the recipe on page 202.

Broccoli slaw: This is basically coleslaw made from broccoli stems rather than cabbage. It's a great low-calorie, satisfying, and volumizing addition to salads, pita sandwiches, and stir-fries. It's tasty warmed up too. Just empty the bag of slaw into a microwave-safe dish and microwave on high for about a minute or two per cup of slaw, then add olive oil and salt and pepper. Or better yet, mix a tablespoon of Cheez Whiz Light in with the slaw. It will melt and taste delicious, just like it did when you were a kid.

Mini seedless cucumbers: These are great for snacking on. Eat as many as you like. They are especially good for when you have the munchies but aren't really hungry, or for when you are cooking and tempted to snack on the foods you're preparing.

Zucchini: So amazingly healthy, and it tastes great just steamed with a little salt and pepper and a touch of grated Parmesan cheese or olive oil.

Sugar snap peas: These aren't peas in the pod and they're not snow peas; you can think of them as a cross between the two. They're low in carbs and super delish to snack on while making dinner. I just eat them raw. Yum!

Celery: With so few calories, why wouldn't you always have celery fresh in the fridge? Dip it in hummus, salsa, fat-free black bean dip, light ranch dip, Cheese Whiz Light—the options are endless.

Tomatoes: Hot house tomatoes are great for slicing on sandwiches; cherry and grape tomatoes are great for throwing into salads. Tomatoes make everything good.

Bean sprouts: These are a must for anyone trying to lose weight. They add loads of volume, crunch, and fiber for virtually no calories. Put handfuls in your salads, stir-fries, wraps, sandwiches, and pitas.

Basil: Buy this fresh and put it in everything from omelets to dressings to pasta sauces.

Mint: Mint leaves add loads of flavor and taste great when torn up and thrown in salads or sandwiches.

Sweet potato: This is a low-calorie root vegetable that is way healthier than its distant relative, the potato. A large sweet potato has only 160 calories and is high in fiber and water, making it filling, nutritious, and great for a lunch, side dish, or snack. Check out my Cheesy Sweet Potato recipe on page 183.

Spaghetti squash: It's amazingly healthy and nutritious, and has only 40 calories per cup cooked. After it's cooked, you just scrape out the strands with a fork to get the spaghetti effect, and then be creative—use it as you would pasta or sweet potatoes. It's even amazing just topped with Becel Topping and Cooking Spray and a dash of cinnamon and sweetener.

Butternut squash: Healthy, high in nutrients, and low in calories—only 60 calories per cup. Butternut squash is ideal for weight loss. You can buy it whole, but most grocery stores also sell it ready to go, peeled and diced. I top it with a tablespoon of olive oil, sprinkle it with rosemary and salt and pepper, and bake it in the oven at 400°F for about 45 minutes until it gets nice and crispy like fries.

Fruits

Apples: Fuji and Royal Gala are my favorites, but feel free to try out any variety that catches your eye. I always

have apples in my fridge. An apple a day does keep the
doctor away. (Don't worry, I won't take offense.)

Berries: Blueberries, strawberries, raspberries, black-
berries—they're all great and super waistline-friendly.
When they're not in season, stock up on the frozen
varieties.

Bananas: Because bananas are slightly high in calories,
I recommend eating half at a time. Slice half into your
cereal or yogurt and then freeze the other half; you can
use it later to make smoothies.

Grapefruit: A delicious snack! Sprinkle it with sweetener mixed with cinnamon for a sweet treat.

Grapes: I recommend eating grapes frozen. They taste
delicious, have a satisfying texture, and take longer to eat.

BULK FOOD, NUTS, AND SEEDS • • • • • • • • • • • • •

Pumpkin seeds: These are super-healthy, but use them
sparingly because they're very high in calories. One or
two tablespoons on a salad is perfect.

Almonds: Slivered almonds add wonderful flavor and
crunch when toasted in the oven and then added to
green beans, salads, and fish.

Pistachios: Yum, yum, yum—about 20 make for a great
snack.

Walnuts: I buy walnuts in pieces and use them in pesto sauce; see page 203 for the recipe. It works well on pasta, of course, but also makes a delicious paste for fish and chicken.

Ground flax seeds: Buy them pre-ground or grind them yourself. Make sure to keep them in an opaque (non-clear) bag and store them in the fridge, otherwise they can go rancid quickly. Add a tablespoon to yogurt, cottage cheese, or cereal for a major omega 3 and fiber punch. They have a nice, nutty flavor, and about 30 calories per tablespoon.

Whole flax seeds: Whole flax seeds are high in soluble fiber, although the omega 3 isn't released unless they're ground up. I add a teaspoon to yogurt or cereal.

DAILY •••••••••••••••••••••••••••••••••••

Milk, Cream, and Eggs
I'm sooo over my lactose intolerance, and I hope you are too (if not, you can use Lactaid). Below are some of my all-time fave dairy products.

Cows' milk: It's always good to have 2%, 1%, or skim on hand. If you don't like milk, you can use soy milk or almond milk instead.

Blue Diamond Almond Breeze: These almond milks are made from filtered water and almonds, so they are not actually a dairy product at all. The unsweetened vanilla and chocolate flavors are unbelievably good, and are some of the best new products I've tested. Almond milk is great with cereal and in smoothies, but I love drinking a cup on its own. It tastes so good and refreshing, and 1 cup has only 40 calories.

Buttermilk: This is great, low in fat, and excellent for soaking chicken in to tenderize and flavor it before cooking.

Cream: Fine, I'll admit it. I like a little half and half in my coffee. Although it's very high in fat, the dose makes the poison, so if you limit yourself to no more than 1 or 2 tablespoons per day, you're okay in my books.

MimicCreme Unsweetened Cream Substitute: This stuff is very interesting. It's a non-dairy cream made from water and almonds, and has only 10 calories per tablespoon. It can be substituted one for one in place of cream in any recipe. If you're trying to avoid dairy, give it a try. Check out www.mimiccreme.com, or find it at www.lowcarbgrocery.com.

Whole Foods 365 Organic Coffee Creamer Natural Vanilla Flavor: This is like Coffee-mate, except it doesn't contain any trans fat. It's great for adding texture and flavor to smoothies; just dissolve 1 tablespoon (30 calories worth) in ¼ cup of warm water, then add it to your smoothie.

Reddi-wip Original Whipped Light Cream: Two tablespoons have only 15 calories. This tastes great on fruit, Jell-O, light ice cream desserts, and smoothies. And best of all, it doesn't contain hydrogenated oil, which is often found in other low-fat brands of whipped cream.

Eggs: Always good to have on hand. I buy the organic omega 3 variety.

Liquid egg whites: These are so convenient, and such a perfect food for weight loss. Three-quarters of a cup has only 100 calories. I dare you to try to eat an omelet that big—that's basically the whole carton! I usually use about a quarter of a cup for a really good-sized omelet, which is only 35 calories or so—ridiculously low. Don't be shy when you pour the egg whites into your frying pan. Oh, and by the way, they're practically all protein. Could there even be a better food? No wonder bodybuilders and athletes eat these like crazy when they're trying to lean out.

Butter and Margarine

Becel Light: Gone is the hydrogenated oil (thank goodness!). Two teaspoons have only 35 calories.

Becel Topping and Cooking Spray: I'll admit it: I *love* this product. Some people may be wary, but…it's basically just water (that's the first ingredient) and trace soybean oil. It has zero calories. I'd much rather put this in my body on occasion than artery-clogging butter or spreads full of trans fats. I use it to add delicious, buttery flavor and moisture to popcorn, corn on the cob, vegetables, and toast.

Gay Lea Light Spreadables *(Canada)*: I really like this product. It's butter made spreadable by adding a small

amount of canola oil. It's lower in calories than regular
butter, is so much easier to spread, and tastes great.

Cheeses and Dips

Laughing Cow Light Swiss Original Cheese: These are
amazing. One wedge is creamy, delicious, and, best of
all, has only 22 calories. I eat these alone as a snack, or
put them fresh or melted on top of salads, sandwiches,
crackers, omelets, and pastas.

Mini Babybel Light Cheese: These cheeses (covered in
red wax, remember?) aren't just for kids anymore. One
cheese has only 50 calories, and two of them make a
nice, protein-packed snack to throw in your lunch bag
for midday.

Light or part skimmed shredded cheese: This is so handy to have on hand to add flavor and protein to omelets
and salads. **Kraft Part Skim Mozzarella** and **Kraft Light
Cheddar** work well—⅓ cup equals 90 calories, which is
enough to add flavor and texture to salads and omelets.

Breakstone's Fat Free or 2% Cottage Cheese: This is *very*
good cottage cheese, and worth looking for. It's usually
sold in supermarkets in Jewish areas in the kosher dairy
section. If you can't find it, you can use any fat-free or low-
fat cottage cheese, such as **Nordica** or **Lucerne** *(Canada).*

Light ricotta cheese: Calabro makes a fat-free ricotta
cheese from skim milk that has only 30 calories per ¼
cup. The next best (and slightly easier to find in *Canada*)
is **Allegro 4% Ricotta**: it has 60 calories per ¼ cup and

tastes so creamy and delicious. Ricotta cheese works well in omelets, on pasta dishes, and in desserts. See page 211 for my delish Pumpkin Cheesecake Dessert using ricotta.

Light cream cheese: Organic Meadow is my favorite light cream cheese. **Philadelphia Light Cream Cheese** is also good.

Light feta cheese: One or two tablespoons crumbled on a Greek salad adds so much flavor that you don't even need an oily dressing. Just use balsamic vinegar and a little feta and you're good to go. **Apetina Light** is a fantastic brand.

Fat-free sour cream: Sour cream is great on sweet potatoes, or as part of a low-calorie cream sauce for pasta dishes. Any brand will do.

Yogurt

Fage 0% Total Yogurt *(US)*: This creamy Greek yogurt is amazing and consistently gets rave reviews. One container (170 grams or 6 ounces) has 90 calories and a whopping 15 grams (0.5 ounces) of protein! This is truly an amazing yogurt.

Dannon Light & Fit Yogurt 60 Calorie Packs *(US)*: Each snack-size container in these packs has only 60 calories, and there are lots of flavors to choose from.

Trader Joe's Low Fat Vanilla Yogurt *(US)*: This is a delicious yogurt that offers a more filling snack option. One container has 180 calories, but is 227 grams (8 ounces), so quite a bit bigger than some of the other yogurt snack containers.

Astro Original Balkan Style Natural Yogourt
(Canada): Yes, it's high in fat (6%), but it tastes *amazing* and is virtually sugar- and carb-free. A half cup has 100 calories, and it's worth it.

Astro Original Fat Free and 1% Plain Yogourt
(Canada): This also tastes great, especially for a yogurt that has virtually no sugar. Half a cup has only 60 calories. I often mix this with the Balkan Style for the best of both yogurt worlds.

Yoplait Source 0% 100 gram single servings *(Canada)*: These are sooo delicious and only have 35 calories per container. Believe it or not, they're actually quite filling due to the protein and gelatin in them. I highly recommended this product, although it does contain a small amount of sucralose. I often mix a container of this with a half cup of fat-free or light cottage cheese or ricotta cheese.

CHAPTER 11

GROCERY AISLES

BEVERAGES •

Most drinks, such as soft drinks and juices, are disasters for weight loss. They pack loads of calories, are nutrient-poor, and tend to increase sugar cravings—the exact opposite of what we want. That being said, some drinks, such as the ones listed below, are a satisfying and refreshing change from plain old water. So drink up!

Tea: We all know how wonderful tea can be for our health and waistline, especially green tea. If you're not a tea lover, give these kinds a try, because they taste pretty darn good: licorice (**President's Choice Licorice Spice Herbal Tea** *(Canada)* is good), jasmine green tea, and **Good Earth Sweet & Spicy Herbal Tea.**

Light hot chocolate: This will totally help you with your chocolate cravings, so get some right now! **Swiss Miss Diet Hot Cocoa** has only 25 calories, and **Carnation Hot Chocolate Light** is similarly low at 45 calories. They are both made with a small amount of Splenda and artificial sweetener (the same sweetener that's used in diet soft drinks, such as Coca-Cola Zero). If you'd prefer to stay natural, you can easily make your own. There is an excellent recipe for homemade, natural hot chocolate using Truvia organic sweetener (35 calories per cup) at www.truvia.com.

Vegetable juices and cocktails: These are great for staving off hunger pangs. They pack loads of nutrition and fiber, and are filling and satisfying, so they're great to have on hand—especially around 4 pm, when many a tummy is growling. My favorite brands are **V8 Vegetable Cocktail, R.W. Knudsen Very Veggie Juice,** and **PC Blue Menu 8-Vegetable Cocktail** *(Canada)*. Buy low sodium varieties if you can.

Flavored waters: Hint Essence Water (all natural, zero calories), **SoNu Water** (organic, 45 calories per cup), and **O.N.E. Coconut Water** (all natural, 60 calories in 325 milliliters (11 fluid ounces)—almost a cup and a half) are all refreshing options. I also love **True Lemon** and **True Lime** packets; I add one or two of these calorie-free packets to water for a delicious, guilt-free, calorie-free lemonade. **Vitamin Water 10** is my absolute favorite; it tastes amazing, has only 25 calories for the whole bottle, and uses my favorite organic sweetener, erythritol. (You can't get this in Canada yet, but I hope it will get here soon!)

Soda water: Contrary to popular belief, soda water is not high in sodium (salt), as the name might suggest. I love soda water and often use it to thin out juices; ¼ cup juice with ¾ cup soda water is delish! I also love **Perrier Lemon** and **Perrier Lime** as well as **PC Blue Menu Soda** *(Canada)*, which has zero calories, multiple flavors, and no sweetener.

FROZEN FOODS •

Packaged Frozen Entrees and Appetizers

Frozen foods have come a long way over the years. No longer are they packed with artificial ingredients and disgusting flavors and textures. In fact, nowadays they can be downright delicious and nutritious. Some of my favorite goodies to pick up in the frozen section are listed here.

Amy's Kitchen: Excellent burritos, frozen entrees, soups, and more. Read through the chapter on Lunches and Dinners in Part Three to see how you can incorporate these meals into a healthy day of eating.

Lean Cuisine: These dishes have come a long way. The Spa line is particularly good; check out the Lunches and Dinners chapter to see my faves.

Health is Wealth Vegetable Spring Rolls: These spring rolls are vegan, but they taste absolutely incredible and are so low in calories—six spring rolls have only 210 calories. I dip them in PC Blue Menu Plum Sauce.

Health is Wealth Veggie Munchees: These are so yummy! They are also vegan and low in calories; six munchees have only 150 calories. Wow!

A.C. LaRocco Bruschetta Style Pizza: If you're craving pizza, this one is a real winner—both in taste and especially in calories. Unlike most pizzas, which pack upwards of 1,000 calories per pizza (and trust me, most gals and guys I know can, and do, eat a full pizza no problem), this one has only 340 calories for the whole thing. It's worth asking your grocer to get this in.

Boca Original or Spicy Chik'n Patties: If you don't eat chicken, or even if you do, try these vegetarian burgers. They're made with soy and have only 160 calories per burger. Also try the **Original Chik'n Nuggets** made with natural ingredients.

Frozen soy beans (edamame): These are a fabulous snack or side dish. They're high in protein and pack about 100 calories in 35 beans, which is equivalent to ½ cup once shelled.

PC Blue Menu *(Canada)*: I'm very impressed with this brand. They have lots of great options for meals, so browse a bit the next time you're shopping in a store that offers President's Choice products. Check out the chapter on Lunches and Dinners in Part Three to see my favorites as well as my suggestions for incorporating them into a day of eating.

Frozen Desserts

The Skinny Cow products: The cones have 150 calories and are totally delish. The ice cream sandwiches are also scrumptious and have only 140 calories. And neither has any artificial sweetener. The Skinny Cow is hot (literally—check her out on the website, www.skinnycow.com).

Breyers 100 Calorie Ice Cream Cups: I love these. They taste amazing and are just the right amount. Have one on its own or top it with berries and light whipped cream.

Diet Snapple on Ice Pops: These popsicles are awesome! Just 15 calories for each and they taste *so* good. Just so ya know, they're sweetened with Splenda.

So Delicious Dairy Free Minis (soy-based ice cream sandwiches): If you don't eat dairy, these are a good option. One sandwich has 90 calories.

Frozen Breakfast Items

Amy's Toaster Pops: Amy's toaster pops—apple or strawberry flavored—can be a great nutritious snack or quick breakfast on a busy day. One pop has 150 calories.

Frozen waffles: Kashi GOLEAN Blueberry Waffles and **Nature's Path Organic Frozen Waffles** are amazing and have only 170 calories for two waffles. My absolute favorite, however, is **Van's 97% Fat Free Waffles** (two waffles have 140 calories). Top them with butter spray, berries, cinnamon mixed with sweetener, light pancake syrup, or even low-fat cottage cheese and cinnamon for a fabulous, healthy breakfast or snack. Experiment and enjoy.

PC Blue Menu Steel-Cut Oats with Wild Blueberries *(Canada)*: Brilliant! Now you can have steel-cut oatmeal in minutes. Just pop this frozen breakfast in the microwave and voilà—a delish meal that can help you lower your cholesterol, while keeping you full and satisfied for hours.

CANNED FOOD AND SOUPS •••••••••••••••••

Soups

Healthy soups are excellent for weight-loss plans because they have very low caloric densities, yet high nutrient densities. Plus, they take a long time to eat and are satisfying and comforting. That's why I've included lots of them in the Lunches and Dinners chapter in Part Three. (When I refer to "soup" in Part Three, I'm referring to a homemade soup that has about 100 calories or one of the soups listed here in a portion size of 100 calories.)

In addition to chicken and vegetable broths and stocks, these are some good soups to have on hand.

Kikkoman Instant Miso Soups: These are so quick and easy, very low in calories, and great as a warm snack or as a side for lunch.

Lipton Cup-a-Soup individual packets: Good flavors are beef vegetable, chicken noodle, and spring vegetable.

Imagine Organic Soups: The microwavable tomato soup is great and very filling as part of an easy lunch. The boxed soups are also great in flavors such as creamy tomato, tomato basil, portobello mushroom, chicken, and broccoli. All are made without dairy and have about 60 to 90 calories per cup.

Amy's Organic Soups: These are amazing and so healthy. I recommend all of them. The black bean, split pea, and lentil soups make a great meal packed full of protein and healthy carbohydrates. The organic chunky vegetable soup, no chicken noodle soup, and organic alphabet soup are great alongside meals because they have fewer calories than the soups with legumes, which are more filling.

Campbell's soups: The varieties I suggest are ready-to-eat Chunky Chicken Vegetable, Southwestern Chicken, and Vegetable Beef; ready-to-eat Soup at Hand Blended Vegetable Medley and Garden Tomato, and condensed Half Fat Cream of Mushroom soup.

Canned Vegetables and Fish

Hearts of palm: So good! Buy them canned and snack on them or cut them up into salads. Make a quick and easy salad with cucumbers, hearts of palm, cherry tomatoes, salt, pepper, and balsamic vinegar.

Pumpkin: Buy canned pure pumpkin such as **Libby's 100% Pure Pumpkin** or **e.d. Smith Pure Pumpkin.** It's low in calories, high in fiber, and great in baking. You can also use it for smoothies, by blending it with vanilla-flavored or plain fat-free yogurt plus cinnamon, nutmeg, sweetener, and crushed ice. Or use it for dips by whipping it with low-fat cream cheese, ricotta, or cottage cheese along with sweetener and pumpkin pie spice. Check out my Pumpkin Cheesecake Dessert on page 211. And feel free to experiment!

Canned tomatoes: A must for whipping up pasta sauces.

Tuna packed in water: My favorite is light tuna packed in water; half the can has only 60 calories or so.

Canned wild salmon: This tastes great and is packed with healthy omega 3 fats and protein. However, it has double the calories that tuna has, so be mindful of portion size.

Manischewitz Gefilte Fish: Ready-to-eat and high in protein and healthy fats, this fish can be a real winner for a quick lunch. Don't be scared—just try it! You can find it in the grocery aisle that has kosher products.

CEREALS AND BAKED GOODS ••••••••••••••

Nature's Path Organic Cereals: Many of these are low in calories because they're puffed full of air. My favorite is the Kamut Puffs (1 cup has only 50 calories and tastes amazing with a little sweetener). Also, try Corn Puffs (1 cup has 60 calories), Millet Puffs (1 cup has 50 calories), and Rice Puffs (1 cup has 50 calories). Arrowhead Mills also makes great puffed cereals that are similarly low in calories.

Multi-Grain Cheerios: One cup has 110 calories and is an excellent cereal that will make you feel like a kid again! I love putting a few tablespoons of Cheerios on top of light yogurt for a nice treat before bedtime.

Bran cereals: This is an interesting category. Most people think that bran products and cereals are inherently super-nutritious, but that isn't always the case. For instance, All-Bran Original (100 calories per cup) is made with high fructose corn syrup; All-Bran Buds (70 calories per ⅓ cup) has sugar as the second ingredient, and Fiber One (120 calories per cup) contains aspartame. If you really love these cereals, I would recommend that you add only a few tablespoons to yogurt or other cereals rather than eating a whole cup at a time. A really good, natural, high-fiber cereal is Kashi GOLEAN, which is made with whole grains and sweetened with evaporated cane juice (1 cup has 140 calories).

Whole Foods 365 Organic Multi-Grain and **Oatmeal: PC Blue Menu** *(Canada)* oatmeal packets are awesome! If you don't mind spending a little more time preparing your steel-cut oats, try **McCann's Irish Oatmeal.**

New Sun Cookies: These all-natural, low-fat cookies are packed with fiber and make a great breakfast on the go. The Sugar-Free Apple Cinnamon and Raisin Bran are my favorites, but I also love the Oatmeal Chocolate Chip. Two cookies washed down with a glass of unsweetened almond milk can really hit the spot.

Vitalicious VitaMuffins and VitaTops: One muffin or muffin top has only 100 calories. Have one or two for breakfast and don't feel guilty for a single minute! Personally, I love the chocolate chip sugar-free muffin tops. They're big and chocolaty—need I say more?

CONDIMENTS, DRESSINGS, SPREADS AND COOKING AND BAKING NEEDS••••••••••••••

These are the products worth stocking in your pantry and fridge, since you'll use them over and over and over.

Sugar Substitutes

There are many sweeteners on the market now that are actually natural, and some are even organic. Gone are

the days when aspartame was your only choice. These
are my favorites.

Truvia: Check out www.truvia.com. This is a combo of
erythritol and rebiana from the stevia leaf. It is natural,
doesn't induce gas, and packs a lot of sweetness.

Erythritol: This non-digestible natural sugar alcohol is
great. You can buy it in packets (**Wholesome Sweeteners
Organic Zero** individual packets) or in bulk (**Sensato
Erythritol Crystals** and **NOW Foods Erythritol**). It's
not as sweet as sugar or Splenda, so you have to use a few
packets to taste the same sweetness.

Just Like Sugar: This is an all-natural calorie-free sweetener based on chicory root dietary fiber. It's quite sweet
and is great mixed with cinnamon.

SweetPerfection: This is also a natural sweetener based
on oligofructose from chicory root. You can use it exactly as you would use sugar in baking.

Dixie Diners' Club Sugar Not: This tastes really, really
good! It's sweeter than sugar so a little goes a long way. It
has zero calories and is all-natural, based on lo han fruit
concentrate.

Agave nectar: My favorite brand is **Wholesome Sweeteners Organic Raw Blue Agave.** This is a delicious
and nutritious alternative to sugar and honey. It has
60 calories per tablespoon, but it has a much lower
glycemic index than either sugar or honey, and you don't
need to use very much at all.

Real maple syrup: This is just so good and sweet, and offers more nutrients than refined sugar. However, it is very high in calories. I dilute mine by using just a little and thinning it out with either unsweetened almond milk or Walden Farms Calorie Free Pancake Syrup.

Walden Farms Calorie Free Pancake Syrup: This is an amazing product. I'm not a huge fan of most light syrups on the market because I find that they have a funny aftertaste or use certain sugar alcohols that induce bloating and gas. However, this product totally surprised the heck out of me by doing neither. It's basically filtered water, maple flavor, and Splenda. It's great added to waffles, French Toast (see my recipe on page 163), yogurt, fruit, and sweet potatoes. Walden Farms products are often in the aisle where Jewish and kosher products are found in your supermarket.

Oils and Cooking Sprays

Flax oil and hemp oil: These are both wonderfully high in omega 3 fatty acids.

Extra virgin olive oil (EVOO): Olive oil is a must. It's great for salad dressings, atop veggies, with whole grain breads, and on pasta dishes. However, even though EVOO is super-healthy, remember that all oil has 9 calories per gram, which means that a mere tablespoon has roughly 120 calories. Watch the amount you use, or the pounds will pack on. Think about this: a tablespoon of oil has more calories than ½ cup of cooked pasta!

Canola oil: I prefer this to olive oil for cooking at high temperatures. Although, truth be told, I try not to fry a lot at high temperatures at all, and prefer to boil, broil, bake, barbecue, and poach instead.

Sesame oil and toasted sesame oil: Yum! The makings of a great salad dressing: 1 tablespoon of toasted sesame oil, 1 tablespoon of rice wine vinegar, 1 tablespoon of soy sauce, and a little sugar or sugar substitute.

Cooking sprays: These are a must for spraying baking sheets and frying pans. My absolute favorite brand is Spectrum, especially **Spectrum Canola Spray Oil**, which is good for high temperature cooking. **PAM** is also a tried and true brand (time for a shout-out to my mom, Pamela—Hi Mom!).

Vinegars and Dressings

Vinegars: Rice wine, balsamic, white wine, and apple cider vinegars are fantastic. They add loads of flavor for virtually no calories. Be careful with balsamic glazes, though; they can contain a ton of sugar, so read the label.

Salad dressings: I usually prefer to make mine at home. However, there are some very good store-bought brands out there. These are my favorites:

- **Maple Grove Farms organic and low calorie salad dressings and vinaigrettes** *(US)*: Try Fat Free Vidalia Onion Dressing, All Natural Maple Fig Dressing, Organic Balsamic Fat Free Vinaigrette, All Natural Sesame Ginger Dressing, and All Natural Ginger Pear Dressing, to name a few. Check out the different varieties, and opt for ones that have fewer than 60 calories for 2 tablespoons.

- **Newman's Own Natural Salad Mists:** They're super-low in calories and contain much healthier ingredients than some of the other salad dressing sprays and mists on the market. **Newman's Own Lighten Up and Low Fat Salad Dressings** are also great. My personal favorite is the Low Fat Thai Sesame (2 tablespoons have 35 calories).
- **Kraft Light Done Right, Free, Fat Free, and Calorie-Wise Dressings:** My personal favorites are Calorie-Wise Coleslaw Dressing (2 tablespoons have 60 calories) and Fat Free Catalina Dressing (2 tablespoons have 50 calories).
- **PC Blue Menu Dressings** *(Canada)*: Great picks are Fat-Free Mango Vinaigrette (2 tablespoons have 30 calories), Fat-Free Raspberry Vinaigrette (2 tablespoons have 20 calories), and Fat-Free California Dressing (2 tablespoons have 40 calories).

Feel free to mix ½ tablespoon olive oil with the vinaigrettes above to dress a large salad. Or use 2 tablespoons of the California or coleslaw dressing and add balsamic or rice wine vinegar to give it more flavor without adding calories.

Note: In Part Three, when I say "light vinaigrette," you should aim to use no more than 100 calories' worth of dressing. Use the ones listed here, or use a maximum of 1 tablespoon of oil—the rest should be vinegar, salt, pepper, and spices.

Condiments and Spreads
Guiltless Gourmet Fat Free Black Bean Dip: Even if you don't like beans, try this. It's so good—flavorful to

the max, nutritious, and so low in calories (2 tablespoons have only 40 calories). Use this as a dip or spread for veggies and crackers, on salads, or on sandwiches.

Cheez Whiz Light: Believe it or not, this actually isn't bad for you. It's basically modified milk ingredients, cheese, and water. It tastes amazing and has only 30 calories per tablespoon. I love it spread on crackers, sandwiches, and celery sticks, or heated in the microwave as a warm cheese sauce for veggies.

Peanut butter: PB is one of my favorite foods in the world. Although it's high in fat and calories, you can still indulge while losing weight if you watch amounts. Opt for one lower in fat, such as **Kraft Light Smooth Peanut Butter,** or go with a healthy nut butter such as organic almond butter (buy it prepared or grind your own at health food stores).

Another option is **Bell Plantation PB2 Powdered Peanut Butter**—a really cool product. It's crushed peanuts, with much of the fat extracted, combined with a little salt and sugar. To make it into peanut butter, you just add 1 tablespoon of water (or unsweetened almond milk) to 2 tablespoons of PB2 powder. It turns into a peanut butter spread that has no added oil, preservatives, or trans fats, like many on the market. Plus, it's way lower in calories than other peanut butters: it has about 50 calories for 2 tablespoons, while most peanut butters (even natural ones) have double that for 1 tablespoon. But it is hard to find. I order the chocolate flavor from www.netrition.com or www.lowcarbgrocery.com. Check out the Bell Plantation website, www.bellplantation.com, for lots of tips and recipes.

Unsweetened applesauce: A few tablespoons is fabulous on sweet potatoes, squash, oatmeal, and cottage cheese, and even alongside meats and chicken. The Whole Foods 365 Organic brand is particularly delish.

Walden Farms Calorie Free Apple Butter: This isn't butter at all; it's really just apple flavor and water with some sucralose. It has zero calories and is kosher—you can probably find it in the kosher section of your grocery store. Try it on sandwiches, sweet potatoes, and squash, or in salad dressings. However, if you don't like the taste or idea of Splenda, you won't like this product.

Kraft Fat Free Mayonnaise: This tastes so good and is wonderful for adding creaminess and flavor, especially to tuna.

Yellow and Dijon mustards: Mustard adds delicious flavor to sandwiches; plus it is healthy, packed with phytonutrients, *and* low in calories.

PC Blue Menu Plum Sauce *(Canada)*: This has great flavor and is an awesome dip, especially for Health is Wealth Vegetable Spring Rolls.

Extracts: Vanilla, lemon, almond, and coconut extract add great flavor to smoothies.

Spices: The more the merrier. What could be better than flavor without calories? Here's a good list to start with: allspice, basil, black pepper, caraway seed, cardamom, cayenne pepper, chili pepper, cinnamon, cumin, garlic powder, kosher salt, nutmeg, oregano, and **Keen's Dry Mustard.**

Frontier Certified Organic Bac'Uns: This is a healthy, vegetarian bacon-bit substitute made from textured vegetable protein. It doesn't have trans fat and is way lower in calories than regular bacon. It adds such awesome crunch to salads that you'll never crave croutons again!

Knox Gelatine: If you're leery of diet Jell-O because of the sweetener, make your own jelly molds using unflavored gelatin, fruit juices, and soda water. Yum!

CRACKERS •

Crackers are just so convenient for a quick snack. Problem is, it's way too easy to overindulge. Although they sound innocent enough, crackers are responsible for the return of many a dieter's fat pants. So if you want crackers, go ahead, but watch portion sizes and choose high fiber options such as the ones listed here.

- **Kavli Crispy Thin Crispbreads:** 1 bread serving equals 6 crackers
- **Multifibre Melba Toast rounds:** 1 bread serving equals 6 crackers
- **Ryvita Light Rye Crispbreads:** 1 bread serving equals 4 crackers
- **Wasa Light Crispbreads:** 1 bread serving equals 4 crackers
- **Streits Whole Wheat Matzos:** 1 bread serving equals 1 sheet
- **GG Scandinavian Bran Crispbreads:** 1 bread serving equals 6 crackers. These are my absolute favorite crackers. They're super-thick, high in fiber, and have only 12 calories per cracker. But they're hard to find.

You can order them at www.locarbu.com *(US)* or
www.lowcarbgrocery.com *(Canada)*.

PASTA AND RICE •

Okay, I know we all have noodles and rice at home, but
these are the best ones to have in your pantry.

Brown rice: It's so healthy, so don't be afraid of it. Just
bring 1 cup of long grain brown rice and 2 cups water
or broth to a boil, and then reduce heat to simmer and
cover for 45 minutes. Voilà! A half cup of cooked brown
rice has about 100 calories, which equals about one serving of bread. Check out page 52 for my rice "sandwich"
suggestion, and www.usarice.com for other recipe ideas.

Quinoa: This is a high-protein whole grain that is tasty
and nutritious. But it is also high in calories: one cup has
a whopping 640 calories! Since it's high in protein and
has a complete set of amino acids, it's great for vegetar-
ians. Half a cup of cooked quinoa with loads of veggies
makes a nice meal full of fiber, protein, and healthy fats.

Pasta: I love pasta. It's cheap, easy, delicious, and so
versatile. **Catelli** and **Nutrition Kitchen** make fabulous
whole wheat, soybean, and flax varieties that are healthier and lower on the glycemic index than regular white
pasta. Half a cup of cooked whole wheat pasta has about
90 calories—that's pretty low. I mean, it's the same as half
a cup of bran cereal, and less than a tablespoon of oil—
craziness, right? But measure it out, because you may
be eating a lot more than half a cup cooked. To make it
even lower in calories, try these next two suggestions.

Dreamfields Pasta: Available at selected stores or on-line at www.dreamfieldsfoods.com, this pasta is made primarily from 100% durum wheat semolina, not whole wheat flour, so it tastes even better than whole wheat pasta. Plus, it contains inulin, a prebiotic, and most of the carbs aren't even digestible. As a result, it is 65 percent lower on the glycemic index than regular pasta. I've tested it on myself, my husband (without him knowing—ha!), and my colleagues, and none of us had any stomach upset at all. (I get nervous when something says non-digestible, although technically that is the definition of fiber: a non-digestible carbohydrate.) We all loved it. Usually, I go half and half: I mix ½ cup of Dreamfields with ½ cup of another whole wheat or plain pasta for the best of both worlds. It's all about compromise, people.

Shirataki noodles: Repeat after me: zero calories. What? In my opinion, these are the next best thing to sex, wine, and chocolate. Seriously, they're probably even better, because there is no guilt associated with them. Indulge in these *calorie-free* noodles to your heart's delight. Shirataki noodles are made from water and glucomannan, a soluble fiber. And did I mention they have zero calories? They're great added to soups and Asian stir-fries. **House Foods** makes amazing shirataki noodles that are mixed with tofu (don't worry, you can't taste it) to give them an even better texture. They come in angel hair, spaghetti, and fettuccini varieties, and one bag has 40 calories. There are tons of recipes on their website, www.housefoods.com. If your grocery store doesn't carry them, ask them to! Or you can get them from www.lo-carbu.com *(US)* or www.lowcarbgrocery.com *(Canada)*. FYI: To prepare them, I simply cut the bag open, dump

them in a strainer, and then rinse them really well with
warm water for about a minute.

SNACKS AND TREATS • • • • • • • • • • • • • • • • • • •

Freeze-dried and bake-dried fruit: These dried fruits
are crunchy and convenient, and nothing's been added
to them. My favorites are **Sensible Foods Crunch Dried
Fruit** and **Bare Fruit 100% Organic Bake-Dried Fuji
Apple Chips,** both of which you can find at many grocery
and health food stores. They add crunch to yogurt, cottage
cheese, and salads, and also make for a sweet and healthy
mid-day snack. Plus, they don't go bad like regular fruit.
Funky Monkey Freeze-Dried Fruit and **Brothers-All-
Natural Fruit Crisps** are also excellent brands.

Brothers-All-Natural Potato Crisps: When freeze-
dried, potatoes become—you guessed it—healthy potato
crisps. Best of all, they have absolutely no oils, no preservatives, and contain only natural ingredients. A whole
bag has only 45 calories!

Orville Redenbacher's 100 Calorie Mini Bags: When
you're craving something crunchy, go ahead and nuke
one of these bags. They're portion controlled so you
won't overdo it. Feel free to mix in a bag of freeze- or
bake-dried apple chips for a salty–sweet treat.

Jerky: Golden Valley Premium Natural Turkey Jerky
(made with no nitrites and from turkey not raised with
hormones) and **The Blue Goose Cattle Company Original Beef Jerky** (organic) are both sooo delish, and can
really hit the spot when you're in a rush.

YummyEarth Organic Lollipops: These are really good! Three lollipops have 70 calories. You can buy them at www.yummyearth.com.

Meringues: These are a great, low-cal dessert because they're essentially egg whites whipped with air and some sugar. **Miss Meringue** is also a good brand that even has a sugar-free variety—13 cookies for 35 calories! They have fiber and protein, and they taste great (the vanilla ones are my favorite). Though these do contain Splenda and some natural sugar alcohol, they don't bother my stomach at all. **President's Choice Imported Meringue Nests** *(Canada)* are a great "crust" or base for fruit salads, yogurt, and whipped toppings. They are big and sweet and have only 60 calories.

No Pudge! Original Fat Free Fudge Brownie Mix: You just mix this with your favorite fat-free vanilla yogurt and bake (in the microwave or the oven), and voilà—a delicious, chewy, fat-free brownie with only 120 calories!

CHAPTER 12

HEALTH AND SPECIALTY FOOD STORE ITEMS

You can find many of these products at sports nutrition and health food stores, or online at sites such as www.lowcarbgrocery.com and www.netrition.com.

PROTEIN POWDERS

If you're running late, don't have time to cook, or are out of groceries, protein powder whipped into a shake can be a real lifesaver. I don't like protein powders that have artificial sweeteners, so I look for ones that are sweetened with natural sweeteners such as stevia, fructose, or natural sugar alcohols. Here are my favorite choices:

- Sisu Whey Protein Isolate
- Healthy 'N Fit 100% Egg Protein Powder in Heavenly Chocolate
- Optimum Nutrition 100% Whey
- Genuine Health proteins+

NUTRITION/PROTEIN BARS

I hate bars! Okay that's not true. I love bars—dancing and socializing in them, that is. As for protein bars, nutrition bars, and meal replacement bars, though, I hate them. Why? Because they're dry, concentrated sources of calories that often pack unhealthy ingredients like sugar, trans fat, and artificial sweeteners. But…they are so convenient! So if you're on the run, and you must hit the "bar," have one that packs a lot of protein to fill you up, not too much sugar, and no gas-inducing sweeteners and artery-clogging hydrogenated oils. These are my top picks.

Chocolite Protein Bars: These taste delicious and really hit the spot! Best of all, they have only 100 calories, so you don't have to dip too far into your calorie savings. These can make a really nice snack or post-workout treat when you're rushed for time. My favorite flavors are Peanut Butter, Triple Chocolate Fudge, and Chocolate Turtle. Also *amazing* are the Chocolite Finally! products. They look like Turtles and taste just as good, I promise. Each "turtle" has only 30 calories.

Doctor's CarbRite Diet Bars: These are scrumptious, but at 190 calories, they're a bit more filling than the Chocolite bars. They have a ton of awesome flavors, and contain no trans fats or artificial sweeteners. My favorite flavors are Toasted Coconut and S'mores. Pick 'em up at www.amazon.com if you can't find them at your sports nutrition store.

BALANCE Bars: These are great. They have no trans fats or artificial sweeteners and they are tasty. They have 200 calories, so they make a good mid-afternoon snack or quick brekkie when on the run.

Clif 20g Protein Builder's Bar: This is a good meal replacement protein bar. One bar has 20 grams (0.7 ounces) of protein and 270 calories, and is very satisfying. One of these with a glass of almond milk can make for a great after-gym meal-in-the-purse when you're rushed for time.

FullBar: The FullBar is great. It's all-natural, it tastes amazing, and it truly is filling. Each bar has 180 calories or fewer, but is actually quite big and satisfying. My favorite flavor is Peanut Butter Crunch. You can find them in the weight-loss section of many pharmacies in the US, or you can order them online. Check out www. fullbar.com.

PART THREE

THE PLAN—THE ROUTE THAT YOU'RE GOING TO TAKE

(...so that you can throw out your fat pants and let the weight loss begin!)

Get ready to freak out, because you're about to see how easy it is to follow this plan and shed pounds. You have the knowledge from Part One, and you have the ingredients from Part Two, so now you just need some help putting it all together. That's what Part Three is all about.

In this part, I will present you with a variety of meal ideas to suit your varied and ever-changing lifestyle. You will find suggestions for home-assembled meals, easy recipes to cook, store-bought ready-to-go meals, restaurant fare, and even fast food suggestions. I understand that no two rebels are alike and that routines change all the time; this is why I've given you so many different options. In other words, no more excuses, you clever rebel, because you now have a plan suitable for any diet challenge or obstacle that comes your merry way. (Think road trips, celebrations, no groceries, no time...)

Here's how it's going to go down. I have provided you with suggestions for breakfasts, lunches, dinners, and snacks. I recommend that you choose a breakfast, a lunch, a dinner, and up to two snacks per day. Plus, I've listed a number of "free" foods and beverages that you can consume whenever you like in addition to your meals. I've also given you sample meal plans to cover those situations when you just can't figure it out yourself. Now you really have no excuses!

The meals are separated into three categories: Black Diamond, Blue Square, and Green Circle.

◆ Black Diamond meals are the lightest and have the fewest calories.

▉ Blue Square meals are slightly more caloric than Black Diamond meals.

● Green Circle meals, although still super-light and healthy, have the most calories.

Eating from all three categories should result in weight loss. You'll have to experiment to determine which category you choose from for what meal. If you've had a Black Diamond breakfast and lunch, you may want to have a Blue Square meal for dinner. If you worked out like a maniac this morning, you may want to choose all Green Circle meals. If you've been off track for a bit and want to shed some pounds quickly, you may want to choose all Black Diamond meals for a few days. It's up to you, but it's important that you figure out how your body responds to the different categories.

Think of it as skiing. If you ski all the black diamond slopes, you may get discouraged or tired out and have to quit early, so sticking with black diamond isn't necessarily the best strategy. If you just ski green circle slopes, though, you may be going too easy on yourself, and you may not see improvement as quickly as you'd like. Bottom line: mix and match, enjoy, and aim for slow, steady results.

CHAPTER 13

SHRINK-A-CIZING BREAKFASTS

BLACK DIAMOND ●

These Black Diamond breakfasts can be used as snacks too. Remember this when you read through the chapter on snack options starting on page 205.

◆ Black Diamond Breakfast #1

High-fiber crackers topped with something delicious is a perfect and lightning-fast way to start the day. As your base, start with one serving of crackers, such as any of the following:

- 5 Kavli Crispy Thin Crispbreads
- 5 Multifibre Melba Toasts rounds
- 4 GG Scandinavian Bran Crispbreads
- 4 Wasa Light Crispbreads
- 4 Ryvita Light Rye Crispbreads
- 1 sheet whole wheat matzo

Then try any of the following outrageously fabulous toppings:

- 2 heaping tablespoons of fat-free cottage cheese—Breakstone's is best, in my opinion, and worth looking for, but any low-fat variety (2% or less) will do—sprinkled with cinnamon alone or cinnamon mixed with sweetener.

*You can eat them cold or heat them in the microwave
for 15 seconds for a delicious twist.*
- 2 tablespoons of low-fat cream cheese or 2 wedges of
  melted Laughing Cow Light Gourmet Cheese Bites,
  with tomato slices
- 2 tablespoons of prepared chocolate PB2
- 1 tablespoon of low-fat cream cheese topped with
  1 tablespoon of Walden Farms Calorie Free Apple
  Butter
- 2 tablespoons of Cheez Whiz Light

◆ Black Diamond Breakfast #2

Start with one bread serving. See page 107 to remind
yourself what constitutes a bread serving, or use any of
the following:

- 2 slices of Weight Watchers 100% Whole Wheat
  Sliced Bread
- 1 slice of Ezekiel 4:9 Sprouted Whole Grain Bread
- ½ whole wheat pita
- 1 La Tortilla Factory Multi Grain Wrap

Top it with any of the following:
- 2 tablespoons of low-fat cream cheese and sliced
  tomato
- 2 tablespoons of Cheez Whiz Light
- Walden Farms Calorie Free Apple Butter
- A light coating of Becel Topping and Cooking Spray,
  topped with up to 1 tablespoon of cinnamon sweetener (for cinnamon toast!)
  *Make cinnamon sweetener by mixing cinnamon and
  your preferred sweetener to taste.*
- 1 single-serving size cottage cheese (113 gram

container—about ¼ cup—of fat-free Breakstone's or
1% Nordica, for instance)
With bread, it is way better to do these in the oven:
set your oven to broil, spread the cottage cheese on,
sprinkle with cinnamon (plus or minus sweetener), and
then broil for a few minutes until the bread gets crispy.
It's amazing—and it will make you realize how great
cottage cheese is warmed up!

◆ Black Diamond Breakfast #3

Start with 70 to 100 calories' worth of yogurt, milk, or
cottage cheese (flip to page 116 for amazing dairy product recommendations), and mix and match with any of
the following:

- ½ cup of berries (fresh, or frozen and defrosted in the
  microwave)
- ½ bag of Sensible Foods Crunch Dried Fruit or a
  handful of Bare Fruit Granny Smith Apple Chips
- 1 tablespoon of ground flax seeds, whole salba seeds,
  or hemp seeds
- 1 tablespoon of toasted slivered almonds
- 2 tablespoons of your fave high-fiber cereal (see page
  130 for suggestions)

◆ Black Diamond Breakfast #4

This is the ultimate breakfast on the run. Grab one of the
goodies below and wash it down with 1 cup of unsweetened almond milk or ½ cup of skim milk:

- 1 Chocolite Protein Bar (you can have any flavor that's
  100 calories or less; there are so many to choose from
  and they're all awesome!)

- 1 New Sun Apple Cinnamon Cookie
- 1 Vitalicious 100 Calorie VitaTop

◆ Black Diamond Breakfast #5

Make a super-healthy, waistline-friendly cereal for breakfast by combining your favorite brand from the following list with either ½ cup of unsweetened almond milk, ½ cup of skim milk, or 1 single-serving size of Yoplait Source 0% yogurt (a 100 gram container has 35 calories). Add sweetener to taste, if you desire.

- 1 cup of Nature's Path Kamut Puffs, Millet Puffs, Corn Puffs, or Rice Puffs
- ½ cup of Fiber One or All-Bran Original cereal
- ½ cup of Multi-Grain Cheerios
- ¼ cup of dry, rolled oats, such as Bob's Red Mill or Quaker
  Believe it or not, you can eat oats dry and uncooked with milk or almond milk for a delicious muesli-type breakfast cereal. Or, if you prefer to be more traditional, add enough water to cover, and put it in the microwave for 45 seconds. Sprinkle a bit of salt on when it's done and mix it with yogurt as above for a delicious, nutritious breakfast.

◆ Black Diamond Breakfast #6

Who doesn't love an omelet in the morning? These ones are made with just egg whites, they taste terrific, and they're excellent for weight loss.

Egg White Omelet

- cooking spray

- ¼ to ½ cup liquid egg whites
- 2 to 3 tbsp skim milk
- salt and pepper
- your choice of herbs, spices, and veggies

Warm a non-stick pan on medium heat and spray with cooking spray. Beat egg whites, milk, and salt and pepper together in a bowl, then pour the mixture into the pan. Let the omelet cook until it starts to bubble, then add the vegetable toppings of your choice, plus something from the following list:

- 2 tbsp shredded light cheese such as part skim mozzarella or cheddar
- 1 tbsp light feta cheese
- 2 Laughing Cow Light Gourmet Cheese Bites

Flip the omelet in half and cook for another minute or so, until set.

◆ Black Diamond Breakfast #7

Give your digestion a break and soak up some nutrients fast with a simple fruit breakfast—but add a little creativity to keep it interesting and tasty.

- 1 whole grapefruit cut in half and sprinkled with cinnamon sweetener
- 1 cup of berries with 2 tablespoons of light coconut milk (yum!)
- half a cantaloupe, half a honeydew, or half a banana with 3 tablespoons of light cottage cheese
  Cottage cheese is oddly delicious warmed up. Try slicing

half a banana (or any other fruit, for that matter) and adding it to the cottage cheese. Sprinkle with cinnamon sweetener and microwave for about 30 seconds or so. Creamy, warm, and delicious!

Baked Apple

- 1 apple
- Becel Topping and Cooking Spray
- 1 tsp cinnamon sweetener

Slice the apple and place it in a microwave-safe bowl. Spray with Becel Topping and Cooking Spray and sprinkle with cinnamon sweetener. Microwave on high for 1 minute. Enjoy as is or with 1 tablespoon of fat-free cottage cheese or light ricotta cheese, or with a Laughing Cow Light Gourmet Cheese Bite (add the cheese halfway through cooking if you want it warm).

◆ Black Diamond Breakfast #8

A high-protein and veggie-packed breakfast is a great way to start the day, not to mention your metabolism. It packs a very low glycemic load, so your blood sugar and insulin levels will remain low, keeping your body in optimal fat-burning mode. Plus, high-protein breakfasts are very satiating, as it takes your body a while to break down all the chemical bonds in the protein. Give these breakfasts a try (feel free to add sliced veggies on the side) and see how you feel. Lean and clean, I'm sure!

- 3 slices of low-fat chicken, turkey, or ham bacon (Piller's Tastes Better than Bacon is a great brand) with 1 cup of V8 Vegetable Cocktail

- 4 slices of Canadian back bacon (such as Schneiders) with 1 cup of V8 Vegetable Cocktail
- 1 hard-boiled egg sprinkled with salt and pepper, with 1 cup of V8 Vegetable Cocktail
- 4 Yves Veggie Breakfast Links with 1 cup of V8 Vegetable Cocktail
- 2 Mini Babybel Light Cheeses with 1 cup of V8 Vegetable Cocktail

Egg Muffin To Go

Have two egg muffins. This recipe should make a dozen muffins.

- 1 small pkg frozen broccoli or spinach (or you can use fresh vegetables instead)
- ¾ cup liquid egg whites
- ¾ cup shredded low-fat cheese
- ¼ cup diced red onion
- ¼ cup diced bell pepper
- pinch of salt, pepper, and dried basil
- cayenne pepper to taste

Preheat the oven to 350°F. Microwave broccoli or spinach on high for 2 to 3 minutes and drain excess liquid. Spray a muffin tin with cooking spray. Combine all the ingredients in a mixing bowl and then divide the mixture evenly between the muffin tins. Bake for 20 minutes, or until egg has set. Feel free to experiment with different vegetables and quantities.

◆ **Black Diamond Breakfast #9**

Even if you're rushed for time, out of groceries, or feeling rebellious and tempted to just skip breakfast all together, don't! At least have a quick, nutritious drink to get your

day, and your metabolism, started. Try these, and you'll
see how easy and delish a breakfast-in-a-cup can be.

- ½ scoop of protein powder (equivalent to about
  50 calories; see page 143 for suggestions) blended with
  1 cup of unsweetened almond milk and a few ice cubes
- 1 cup of frozen berries blended with 1 cup of
  unsweetened almond milk, sweetener to taste,
  and calorie-free extracts (try vanilla first, then
  experiment)

Iced Vanilla Rebelccino

- 1 tbsp powdered organic coffee creamer, vanilla flavor
- ¾ cup unsweetened vanilla almond milk
- 1 tsp instant coffee
- ¼ tsp vanilla extract
- 2 or 3 packets of Wholesome Sweeteners Organic
  Zero sweetener (or any other sweetener of your
  choice)
- 5 ice cubes
- Reddi-wip Whipped Light Cream (optional)

Dissolve the coffee creamer in 3 tablespoons of warm
water. Add all ingredients to a blender, and blend until
smooth. If you like, top the whole thing with Reddi-wip
Whipped Light Cream. IT'S SO GOOD!

BLUE SQUARE •

▧ Blue Square Breakfast #1

Double the portion size of any Black Diamond breakfast. For example, instead of 1 hard-boiled egg, have 2;
instead of 1 Vitalicious 100 Calorie VitaTop, have 2;
instead of 1 slice of toast with cream cheese and tomato,
have 2.

■ Blue Square Breakfast #2

Combine two different Black Diamond breakfast suggestions. For example, have a hard-boiled egg *and* a slice of toast with cream cheese and tomato. Or have an Egg White Omelet with 4 slices of Canadian bacon.

■ Blue Square Breakfast #3

Start with either one bread serving or one serving of high-fiber crackers, and add any of the following toppings:

- 2 to 3 slices of smoked salmon or lox (about 100 grams or 3 ounces worth), 1 tablespoon of low-fat cream cheese, and sliced tomatoes, cucumbers, onions, and capers
- 1 tablespoon of light peanut butter or a natural nut butter such as almond butter
- 2 tablespoons of prepared PB2 with half a sliced banana
- Make a BLT by adding 1 tablespoon of light mayo, 2 slices of Piller's Tastes Better than Bacon (or any lean chicken, turkey, or ham bacon), lettuce leaves, and sliced tomato

■ Blue Square Breakfast #4

Eggs are super-healthy and packed with awesome protein. The whites are protein and water; the yolks are fat and nutrients. When you buy omega 3 eggs, the yolks pack healthy omega 3 fatty acids. The difference between a Black Diamond omelet and a Blue Square omelet is that now you can add a yolk. Yay, yellow! Yes, it adds a few more calories and fat grams, but it's also more filling.

Egg White and Yolk Omelet

- 1 egg
- 2 egg whites
- 2-3 tbsp skim milk
- salt and pepper
- 3 tbsp of shredded light cheese or 2 Laughing Cow Light Gourmet Cheese Bites
- arugula

Warm a non-stick pan on medium heat and spray with cooking spray. Beat the egg and whites, milk, and salt and pepper together in a bowl, then pour the mixture into the pan. Let the omelet cook until it starts to bubble, then add the cheese. Flip the omelet in half and cook for another minute or so, until set. Serve on a bed of arugula.

■ Blue Square Breakfast #5

Take the light fruit breakfast concept and make it last a little longer with some protein.

- 1 apple with 30 grams (1 ounce) of cheddar cheese or 1 slice of light havarti cheese
- 1 small banana with 1 tablespoon of light peanut butter or natural nut butter

Baked Apple with Nuts

- 1 apple
- Becel Topping and Cooking Spray
- 1 tsp cinnamon sweetener
- 2 tbsp slivered almonds

Slice the apple and place it in a microwave-safe bowl. Spray with Becel Topping and Cooking Spray and sprinkle with cinnamon sweetener and almonds. Micro-wave on high for 1 minute. Enjoy as is or with 1 table-spoon of fat-free cottage cheese or light ricotta cheese, or with a Laughing Cow Light Gourmet Cheese Bite (add the cheese halfway through cooking if you want it warm).

■ Blue Square Breakfast #6

These shakes and smoothies have some extra ingredients to keep your tummy full and your taste buds happy. Toss all the ingredients listed under each option into your blender and blend until smooth.

Berry Wake-Up
- 1 scoop protein powder (equivalent to about 100 calories)
- ½ cup frozen berries
- ½ cup skim milk or unsweetened almond milk
- a few ice cubes

Banana Wake-Up
- ½ scoop protein powder (equivalent to about 50 calories)
- 2 tsp flax oil
- ½ frozen or fresh banana
- ½ cup skim milk or unsweetened almond milk
- a few ice cubes

Iced Mocha
- ½ scoop protein powder (equivalent to about 50 calories)
- ½ cup brewed strong coffee

- 2 tsp flax oil
- 1 tsp low-fat organic coffee creamer dissolved in 2 tbsp warm water
- 2 tsp unsweetened cocoa
- ½ cup skim milk or unsweetened almond milk
- a few ice cubes

Blue Square Breakfast #7

Here are some fantastic prepackaged/restaurant/store-bought breakfasts (McDonald's even!) that are so skinni-mizing, they can still count as Blue Squares.

- 1 Amy's Apple Toaster Pop or Strawberry Toaster Pop
- Amy's Cream of Rice Hot Cereal Bowl
- McDonald's Fruit 'n Yogurt Parfait
- Tim Hortons Low Fat Yogurt with Berries
- PC Blue Menu Steel-Cut Oats with Wild Blueberries (you'll find it in the frozen section of any grocery store that carries President's Choice products)
- 1 packet PC Blue Menu Multi-Grain Instant Oatmeal (or your favorite multigrain oatmeal averaging about 150 to 200 calories) made with water and topped with 2 tablespoons of skim milk or unsweetened almond milk
- Starbucks Perfect Oatmeal with the brown sugar topping
- 2 Nature's Path Organic Frozen Waffles or Van's 97% Fat Free Waffles (topped with butter spray, Walden Farms Calorie Free Apple Butter, or Walden Farms Calorie Free Pancake Syrup)
- 1 BALANCE Bar (any flavor that is 200 calories or less) with 1 cup of unsweetened almond milk
- 1 Doctor's CarbRite Diet Bar (choose any flavor that

is 200 calories or less; S'mores and Toasted Coconut
are my favorites!) with 1 cup of unsweetened almond
milk
- 1 FullBar (any flavor) with 1 cup of unsweetened
almond milk

■ Blue Square Breakfast #8

When the weekend comes and you have a little more
time to prep breakfast and experiment in the kitchen (or
are in a panic to prepare something impressive for your
unexpected overnight guest), try one of these.

French Toast

- ¼ to ½ cup liquid egg whites
- a dash of skim milk or unsweetened vanilla almond
milk
- cooking spray
- 3 slices of low-calorie bread (try Weight Watchers
100% Whole Wheat Sliced Bread)
- Becel Topping and Cooking Spray
- cinnamon sweetener

Heat a non-stick pan over high heat and spray with
cooking spray. Beat the egg whites and milk together
and pour into a shallow dish. Dip the bread slices in the
egg wash one at a time, and fry them, flipping after the
first side has browned (about a minute or so). The bread
should get crispy. Once done, spray the French toast with
Becel Topping and Cooking Spray and sprinkle with
cinnamon sweetener. You can also add Walden Farms
Calorie Free Pancake Syrup on top. Yum!

Fried Matzo

Break 2 sheets of matzo into bite-size pieces and soak in cold water for a minute or so to soften. Pat it dry on paper towels, then prepare it as you would French toast, using the recipe above. It also tastes great savory, using salt and pepper instead of cinnamon sweetener and dipped in a little ketchup.

Kamut Crispy Squares

- 3 tbsp light butter (try Gay Lea Light Spreadables)
- 3 cups mini marshmallows
- 5 cups Nature's Path Kamut Puffs
- 2 cups All-Bran Original Cereal
- cooking spray
- ¼ cup dark chocolate chips

Melt butter in a large skillet or wok over low heat. Stir in marshmallows, and continue stirring until melted. Remove pan from heat. Mix in Kamut Puffs and All-Bran until the cereal is all ooey, gooey, and coated with the marshmallow mixture. Spray a 9″ × 13″ baking pan with cooking spray, and press the cereal mixture in with a spatula. Press chocolate chips randomly into the cereal mixture. Place the pan in the fridge for 20 minutes, until cool, and then cut into approximately 12 squares. Feel free to have 2 squares. These are awesome!

GREEN CIRCLE •

● Green Circle Breakfast #1

Double the portion size of a Black Diamond breakfast, and then combine it with another Black Diamond. For

example, have 2 hardboiled eggs with 1 bread serving, or
have 1 full cup of Multi-Grain Cheerios with an apple.

⬤ Green Circle Breakfast #2
Combine a Black Diamond breakfast with a Blue Square
breakfast. For instance, have 3 slices of turkey bacon
with an Egg White and Yolk Omelet; a grapefruit with
French Toast, or 2 frozen waffles with half a banana and
3 tablespoons of fat-free cottage cheese.

⬤ Green Circle Breakfast #3
Even bigger shakes and smoothies! Toss all the ingredients listed into your blender and blend until smooth.

Strawberry Banana
- 1 scoop vanilla or plain protein powder (equivalent to
  about 100 calories)
- ½ cup frozen strawberries
- ½ frozen banana
- ½ cup skim milk or unsweetened almond milk
- 2 tsp flax or hemp oil
- a few ice cubes

Orange Dream
- 1 scoop vanilla or plain protein powder (equivalent to
  about 100 calories)
- 2 tsp flax oil
- ½ cup orange juice
- ½ cup pineapple pieces
- ½ cup frozen raspberries
- a few ice cubes

Chocolate Banana

- 1 scoop vanilla, chocolate, or plain protein powder (equivalent to about 100 calories)
- 2 tsp flax oil
- ½ cup unsweetened vanilla or chocolate almond milk
- ½ frozen banana
- 2 tsp unsweetened cocoa powder
- a few ice cubes

● Green Circle Breakfast #4

Here are even more nutritious, simple and waistline-loving prepackaged/store-bought breakfasts for you.

- 3 Nature's Path Organic Frozen Waffles or Van's 97% Fat Free Waffles (topped with butter spray, Walden Farms Calorie Free Apple Butter, or Walden Farms Calorie Free Pancake Syrup)
- Clif 20g Protein Builder's Bar with 1 cup of unsweetened almond milk
- Tim Hortons Low Fat Blueberry or Low Fat Cranberry Muffin
- McDonald's Egg McMuffin
- McDonald's Breakfast Burrito
- Starbucks Perfect Oatmeal with the brown sugar topping and either the nut medley or the dried fruit topping

● Green Circle Breakfast #5

I know—this is so easy, it's feeling too good to be true, but it's not! Just to prove it, here are a couple of things you can order at almost any restaurant that will still fit with your plan.

- Smoked salmon platter: Eat only half the bagel (offer the other half to your annoyingly skinny friend, or just spill coffee on it so that you can resist) and opt for light cream cheese (if available). Ask for extra tomatoes, cucumbers, and onions.
- Vegetable egg-white omelet: Even if it's not on the menu, ask for the omelet with egg whites only, light on the cheese. Avoid the deadly home fries; ask for a side salad or tomato slices instead. You can even enjoy this breakfast with 1 slice of lightly buttered whole grain toast.

CHAPTER 14

SKINNI-MIZING LUNCHES AND DINNERS

BLACK DIAMOND •

◆ Black Diamond Lunch or Dinner #1
Have any of the Green Circle breakfasts (starting on page 165) for lunch or dinner.

◆ Black Diamond Lunch or Dinner #2
How 'bout a frozen entrée for a healthy meal in seconds? You can check out page 125 for suggestions, but any entrée with fewer than 300 calories will work. PC Blue Menu, Amy's Kitchen, and Lean Cuisine Spa are all brands I recommend. Here are some examples of awesome dishes that fit the bill.

Lean Cuisine Spa frozen entrées
Mango Curry Chicken; Chicken Mediterranean; Creamy Chicken Alfredo; Chicken in Peanut Sauce; Chicken Caesar Primavera; Grilled Chicken Primavera; Chicken Teriyaki Stir-fry; Wild Salmon with Basil; Thai Chicken; Oven Roasted Beef Burgundy

Amy's Kitchen frozen foods

Brown Rice, Black-Eyed Peas & Veggies Bowl; Teriyaki Bowl; Bean & Cheese Burrito; Bean & Rice Burrito; Black Bean & Vegetable Burrito; Indian Samosa Wrap; Teriyaki Wrap; Garden Vegetable Lasagna; Mexican Tamale Pie; Indian Mattar Tofu Meal; Indian Palak Paneer Meal; Broccoli & Cheese in a Pocket Sandwich; Spinach Feta in a Pocket Sandwich; Spinach Pizza in a Pocket Sandwich; Tofu Scramble in a Pocket Sandwich; Veggie Loaf Whole Meal

PC Blue Menu frozen entrées (*Canada*)

Barley Risotto with Herbed Chicken; Chicken Bangkok; Chicken Tikka Masala; Ginger-Glazed Chicken or Salmon; Linguine with Shrimp Marinara; Parmesan Chicken; any of the "en Papillote" selections

◆ Black Diamond Lunch or Dinner #3

Soup and Sandwich Special! Have any soup you like (go to page 128 for some suggestions, or make your own), as long as it's roughly a 100 calorie portion. Then add one of the sandwich ideas listed below. See page 107 to remind yourself what constitutes a bread serving, or choose one of these options:

- 2 slices of Weight Watchers 100% Whole Wheat Sliced Bread
- 1 slice of Ezekiel 4:9 Sprouted Whole Grain Bread
- ½ whole wheat pita
- 1 La Tortilla Factory Multi Grain Wrap

Deli Sandwich

- 1 bread serving
- 100 g (3.5 oz) deli meat (about 4 slices)
- a few lettuce leaves
- tomato and cucumber slices
- mustard to taste

Start with 1 bread serving, then pile on your favorite deli meat—either lean turkey, ham, or chicken. Add lettuce, tomato, cucumber, and mustard to your liking.

■ To make this into a Blue Square meal, double the amount of deli meat (about 200 grams or 7 ounces).
● To turn this into a Green Circle meal, use 200 grams of deli meat and add an extra bread serving.

Tuna Sandwich

- ⅓ cup (about half a can) canned tuna packed in water, drained
- 1 tbsp fat-free mayo
- mustard to taste
- 1 bread serving
- tomato and cucumber slices (as much as you'd like)

Mix tuna and mayo in a small bowl. Spread mustard on the bread, then pile on the tuna along with tomato and cucumber slices.

■ To make this into a Blue Square meal, use a full can (about ⅔ cup) of tuna.
● To make this into a Green Circle meal, use a full can of tuna and add an extra bread serving.

Egg Salad Sandwich
- 1 hard-boiled egg
- 2 hard-boiled egg whites
- 1 tbsp low-fat mayo
- salt and pepper
- 1 bread serving
- cucumber slices (as much as you'd like)

Make the egg salad by chopping up the hard-boiled egg and egg whites and mixing them in a small bowl with mayo and salt and pepper to taste. Spread it on the bread, and finish the sandwich with cucumber slices and condiments of your choice. Dijon mustard works great!

■ To turn this into a Blue Square meal, double the amount of egg salad by using two whole eggs and four egg whites.

● To turn this into a Green Circle meal, double the egg salad and add an extra bread serving.

◆ Black Diamond Lunch or Dinner #4
How does half a whole wheat pita dipped in lentil soup sound for lunch? How about a slice of hearty whole grain bread alongside a bowl of beef and barley soup? If your answer was "Yum!" give this idea a try.

Pair up any delicious soup (equivalent to about 200 calories) with a bread serving. (Check out the list of Free Foods on page 212 to see what you can add to jazz up your bread.) If you're ordering soup at a restaurant, opt for a broth-based, not cream-based, soup. Soups and chilies that are hearty and packed with beans, lentils, rice, or noodles typically fall in this category. Lentil soup, beef and barley, or split pea would be good choices. A bowl of vegetarian chili would also work. Here are some restaurant options that fit:

- Au Bon Pain: medium bowl of vegetarian chili
- Cosi: 1 regular cup of Moroccan Lentil Soup or Three Bean Chili

Here are a couple of recipes for super-fantastic soup and bread combos.

"Creamy" Protein-Packed Tomato Soup

- 2 cans Campbell's Condensed Tomato Soup (low sodium, if you like)
- ½ pkg of silken tofu, drained (about 175 g or 6 oz)
- ½ cup chopped fresh basil (or 1 tsp dried basil)
- 1 cup water
- 3 tbsp grated Parmesan cheese
- 6 Multifibre Melba Toast rounds

Pour the soup into a blender along with the tofu, basil, and water. Blend until smooth, then pour into a medium saucepan. Cook, stirring frequently, on medium heat until heated through. Pour yourself a 1 cup portion, sprinkle Parmesan cheese into the soup, and crumble Melba Toast Rounds on top. Feel free to swap the crackers with any other bread serving you choose. Store the leftover soup in a jar in the fridge (you should get approximately 3 more servings).

French Onion Soup

- 1 bowl packaged or homemade onion soup, prepared
- 2 slices Weight Watchers 100% Whole Wheat Sliced Bread
- 1 slice light havarti cheese

Pour your soup into an ovenproof bowl. Toast two slices
of bread and crumble them into the soup. Preheat your
oven's broiler, place the cheese on top of the soup, and
slide the soup under the broiler until the cheese is melty
and golden. Voilà! (If you don't have an ovenproof bowl,
skip the broiler for the sake of your dishes. Use a microwave-safe bowl, and simply microwave the soup until the
cheese melts.)

◆ Black Diamond Lunch or Dinner #5

I love sandwiches for lunch and dinner, both on the go
and at home. Here are some quick and easy ways to get a
healthy, filling meal, no matter where your day has taken
you. Sorry ladies, but with options like these, you have
no more excuses for falling off the weight-loss-wagon,
even when you're running around, multitasking like
nobody's business. You go go go girl!

- Subway Mini Sub: Choose a turkey, ham, veggie delite, or chicken Mini Sub (a 4 inch sub). Pile it up with
  unlimited veggies, 1 or 2 cheese slices, and light mayo,
  honey mustard, barbecue sauce, or sweet onion sauce.

■ To turn this into a Blue Square meal, add a bag of
Baked Lay's chips or a side soup of the day (so long as
it's not cream-based).

● To turn this into a Green Circle meal, have a side
order of chili (if your local Subway carries it).

- Subway 6 inch sub: Have a turkey, ham, or veggie
  delite 6 inch sub **without** cheese, and then fill it up
  with unlimited veggies and a little light mayo, honey
  mustard, barbecue sauce, or sweet onion sauce.

■ To turn this into a Blue Square meal, just add cheese.
● To turn this into a Green Circle meal, add cheese and have a side soup of the day (as long as it's not cream-based) or a bag of Baked Lay's chips.

- McDonald's Snack Wrap: If you can find them at your local McD's, try a Snack Wrap—choose either Grilled Chicken, Grilled Caesar Chicken, or Grilled Chipotle Chicken *(Canada)*, or either Chipotle BBQ with Grilled Chicken, Ranch with Grilled Chicken, or Honey Mustard with Grilled Chicken *(US)*. Have a Side Garden Fresh Salad or a V8 (or both) alongside, if you wish.

- Tim Hortons Chicken Wrap Snacker *(Canada)*: Grab either a BBQ Chicken, Chicken Salad, or Chicken Ranch Wrap Snacker and a soup (only choose broth-based soups—no creamy ones).

■ To turn this into a Blue Square meal, have two Wrap Snackers and skip the soup.
● To turn it into a Green Circle meal, have two Wrap Snackers and the soup.

Homemade Chicken Wrap
- 1 large multigrain tortilla (about 100 calories), such as La Tortilla Factory Multi Grain Wraps
- 1-2 tbsp salsa
- 1 tbsp fat-free sour cream
- 1 113 g (4 oz) grilled chicken breast (approximately), sliced, or ⅓ bag Lilydale Fully Cooked Sliced Chicken Breasts *(Canada)*
- loads of shredded lettuce

Spread salsa and sour cream down the middle of the tortilla. Put the chicken and as much shredded lettuce as you can fit on top, and wrap it all up. If you haven't mastered the technique yet, the tortilla package should give you some guidance.

█ To turn this into a Blue Square meal, add 3 tablespoons of shredded part skimmed cheddar cheese.

Stuffed Greek Pita

- ½ whole wheat pita
- 2 tbsp hummus (light, if possible)
- chopped lettuce
- shredded carrots
- cucumber slices
- bean sprouts
- 1 tbsp sunflower seeds

Spread the hummus inside the pita, then stuff the pita with as much chopped lettuce, shredded carrots, cucumber slices, and bean sprouts as you can fit in there, plus the sunflower seeds.

█ To turn this into a Blue Square meal, use ¾ of the pita by cutting away the top quarter so that you can fill it up, and add an extra tablespoon of hummus.

Stuffed Tuna Pita

- ⅓ cup (about half the can) canned tuna packed in water, drained
- 1 tbsp light mayo
- salt and pepper

- ½ whole wheat pita
- ½ apple cut into slices
- shredded carrots
- bean sprouts
- cucumber slices

In a small bowl, mix the tuna with the mayo and salt and pepper to taste. Scoop it into the pita along with the apple slices and then add as many shredded carrots, bean sprouts, and cucumber slices as you'd like.

■ To turn this into a Blue Square meal, use ¾ of the pita by cutting away the top quarter, and use a full can of tuna (⅔ cup) instead of half a can.

◆ Black Diamond Lunch or Dinner #6
Below are some awesome ideas for satisfying lunches and dinners that taste great, pack loads of nutrients, and will keep you full for hours due to the protein content and fibrous, water-packed veggies. Some of these salads taste so good, it's a shame they're even called salads. Think of them as "lettuce cakes" instead!

McDonald's
McDonald's has introduced some awesome tasting (well, that's not a shock), nutritious and low-calorie meal items to their menu. Feel free to try out any of these salad ideas:
- Garden Fresh Salad with Warm Grilled Chicken dressed with 1 packet of Renée's Balsamic Vinaigrette, Mediterranean Greek Dressing.

- Bacon Ranch Salad with Grilled Chicken dressed with 1 packet of Newman's Own Low Fat Balsamic Vinaigrette *(US)*
- Mediterranean Salad with Warm Grilled Chicken dressed with 1 packet of Renée's Mediterranean Greek Dressing *(Canada)*
- Spicy Thai Chicken Salad with Warm Grilled Chicken dressed with 1 packet of Renée's Ravin' Raspberry Dressing *(Canada)*

Subway

Order a large Subway salad with either chicken, tuna salad, turkey, or ham, and dress it with either fat-free Italian or sweet onion dressing. Feel free to ask for a double portion of turkey, chicken, or ham. You can add a Subway soup of the day as well, so long as it's not cream-based.

◼ To turn this into a Blue Square meal, have a bag of Baked Lay's chips or a piece of fruit on the side.

Chicken or Shrimp Greek Salad

You can make this at home, or you can order it in most restaurants. If you're at a restaurant, regular feta cheese is fine, but stick to about 3 tablespoons. Ask for the feta on the side so you can portion it yourself, or if you forget, just leave the rest on your plate—you couldn't possibly have room for another bite!

- mixed lettuce (as much as you want)
- ½ cup (or so) diced tomato
- ¼ cup (or so) sliced onion
- ½ cup (or so) diced cucumbers

- ¼ cup crumbled light feta cheese
- 115 g to 140 g (4 to 5 oz) grilled chicken breast or
  4 large grilled shrimp
- ¼ cup balsamic vinegar (or to taste)

Toss the mixed lettuce, tomato, onion, cucumbers, and feta in a large bowl. Add the chicken or shrimp, and dress the salad with balsamic vinegar. Skip the oil—the cheese adds enough salt, flavor, and fat.

To turn this into a Blue Square meal, replace the balsamic vinegar with 2 tablespoons of your favorite oil and vinegar dressing—but no more!

Chicken Caesar Salad

I know! Isn't this totally illegal on ANY diet? Not on this one. If you're ordering in a restaurant, give the croutons a pass; they tend to be calorie-soaked. Also, order the dressing on the side, so you can dip your fork in the dressing then into the salad, using as little as possible, rather than pouring it on top. Caesar dressing is so full of flavor that just a little can really go a long way. You'll probably enjoy the salad just as much. You'll love it that much more when you notice your pants getting looser.

- 2 cups romaine lettuce (or as much as you want)
- 2 tbsp grated Parmesan cheese
- 1 grilled 140 g (5 oz) chicken breast
- 1 tbsp anchovies (optional)
- 2 tbsp low-fat Caesar dressing

Wash and tear up enough romaine lettuce to create a substantial bed in your bowl. Sprinkle the Parmesan cheese on top, then add the chicken breast and anchovies (if you like them). Add the Caesar dressing and toss to combine.

■ To turn this into a Blue Square meal, add 3 strips of chicken bacon, crumbled, or 3 tablespoons of Frontier Certified Organic Bac'uns on top.

Bean and Seed Salad
- mixed greens
- ½ cup cooked or canned chickpeas
- ½ cup cherry tomatoes
- ½ cup diced cucumber
- ½ cup sliced onion
- 1 tbsp pumpkin seeds
- light vinaigrette or dressing (see page 131 for great options)

Pile up a bed of your favorite mixed greens, then add the chickpeas, tomatoes, cucumbers, onions, and pumpkin seeds. Toss with the vinaigrette or dressing.

Cobb Salad
- romaine lettuce (as much as you want)
- 8 (or so) cherry tomatoes
- ¼ cup crumbled blue cheese
- 1 chopped hard-boiled egg
- 2 chopped hard-boiled egg whites
- ¼ avocado, sliced
- balsamic vinegar or Walden Farms Calorie Free Dressing (or see page 131 for more dressing ideas)

In a big bowl, combine lettuce, tomatoes, cheese, eggs, and avocado. Add dressing and toss.

■ To turn this into a Blue Square meal, add 113 grams (4 ounces) of lean deli meat for an extra protein kick.

Warm Asian Chicken Salad

- 1 tbsp sesame oil
- 1 tbsp low sodium soy sauce
- 1 tbsp rice wine vinegar
- 1 tbsp sweetener such as Just Like Sugar, Sugar Not, or agave nectar
- chopped iceberg lettuce (as much as you like)
- baby spinach (as much as you like)
- ½ cup (or so) bean sprouts
- 8 (or so) cucumber slices
- 15 (or so) snow peas
- cooking spray
- 1 140 g (5 oz) chicken breast, sliced
- ½ cup (or so) water chestnuts, drained

Whisk together sesame oil, soy sauce, rice wine vinegar, and sweetener in a small bowl to combine. Set aside. Heat a skillet on high and liberally coat it with cooking spray. Stir-fry the chicken breast until browned, then pour the sesame dressing in along with the water chestnuts. Sauté for a few minutes more until the chicken is cooked through but the water chestnuts are still nice and crunchy. Put lettuce, spinach, bean sprouts, cucumber, and snow peas in a large bowl. Add the chicken, water chestnuts, and sauce to the salad and toss until mixed. Seriously—YUM!

■ To turn this into a delicious Blue Square meal, add 3 tablespoons of chopped peanuts to the salad.

Fave Fish Dinner

A lovely piece of steamed, baked, or grilled lean fish (such as cod, tilapia, halibut, or tuna steak) and a side of steamed, sautéed, or grilled vegetables makes for a delish, nutrish lunch or dinner anytime, anywhere. If you order it in a restaurant, stick to the fish and vegetable combo, but if you're cuddled up at home, feel free to add 1 slice of hearty whole grain bread or ½ cup of cooked couscous or brown rice. (Fish and veggies tend to be more caloric in restaurants because more oil is used in cooking.)

Manischewitz Gefilte Fish

Have 3 pieces of the fish along with a side salad of mixed greens and vegetables with a light dressing for a great omega 3–packed lunch. The gefilte fish may look…well, gross…but it tastes pretty darn good and is so easy to keep at work or at home in the fridge for a quick, lean protein, ready to go anytime.

◆ Black Diamond Lunch or Dinner #7

If you love carbs—and seriously, I've yet to meet a gal who doesn't—you're going to love these options. Trust me: despite their scary, seriously high-calorie-sounding names, they're actually super waistline-friendly and just the thing this doctor is ordering up.

Pasta Salad

- ½ cup cooked whole wheat penne or Dreamfields penne
- diced cucumbers (as much as you want)
- diced bell pepper (as much as you want)
- diced raw broccoli florets (seriously—as much as you want)
- sliced mushrooms (go nuts!)
- ½ cup diced tomato
- ¾ cup fat-free or 1% cottage cheese
- salt and pepper

Rinse cooked pasta with cold water and drain. Toss pasta, vegetables, and cheese together in a large bowl, and season with salt and pepper to taste. So simple, so good!

■ To turn this into a Blue Square meal, add 3 tablespoons of cooked or canned chickpeas.
● To turn this into a Green Circle meal, use a full cup of penne and add 3 tablespoons of chickpeas.

Cheesy Sweet Potato

- 1 sweet potato
- ½ cup fat-free cottage cheese or 2 Laughing Cow Light Gourmet Cheese Bites
- 1-2 tbsp chives
- salt and pepper

Using a fork, pierce a few holes in the skin of the sweet potato. Wrap it in a paper towel and cook it in the

microwave for 7 minutes on high. Cut it in half, then top
it with the cheese, chives, and salt and pepper to taste.

■ To turn this into a Blue Square meal, crumble 3 slices
of turkey or chicken bacon on top. Another option for a
great Blue Square meal is a Wendy's Hot Stuffed Baked
Potato topped with chives, broccoli, and 3 ounces of
chili.

Simple Tuna Noodle Salad
Try this one in the summer for lunch.
- 1 pkg tofu shirataki or plain shirataki noodles, any
  shape
- ½ cup canned tuna packed in water, drained
- 1 tbsp olive oil
- 2 tbsp grated Parmesan cheese
- salt and pepper

Prepare shirataki noodles according to package directions or just rinse them with warm water followed by
cold water (since this a cold salad), then pat them dry.
Mix noodles with tuna, olive oil, and Parmesan cheese in
a bowl, and season with salt and pepper to taste.

Asian Tilapia on Angel Hair Pasta
- 2 tbsp balsamic vinegar
- 2 tbsp Newman's Own Low Fat Thai Sesame Dressing or Newman's Own Lighten Up Low Fat Sesame
  Ginger Dressing
- 1 tilapia fillet
- 1 pkg angel hair tofu shirataki or plain shirataki
  noodles

- cooking spray
- ½ cup sliced water chestnuts, drained
- a few onion slices
- ½ cup (or so) diced asparagus
- ½ cup (or so) diced bell pepper
- salt and pepper

Whisk the balsamic vinegar and dressing together in a small bowl. Place tilapia fillet in a shallow dish or freezer bag, and pour vinegar and dressing on top. Marinate, refrigerated, for about half an hour.

Preheat oven to 450°F. Make the shirataki noodles according to package directions, or simply rinse well with hot water and pat dry. Set aside.

Tear a piece of aluminum foil into an 8" × 12" rectangle and coat with cooking spray. Place the fish on the foil and add the water chestnuts, onion, asparagus, and bell pepper, then sprinkle salt and pepper to taste on top. Fold the foil into a sealed packet and bake for 20 minutes, or until fish is cooked through. Place the fish and vegetables over the noodles and serve. Delish in a dish!

■ To turn this into a Blue Square meal, use ½ cup of brown rice instead of the shirataki noodles.

● To turn this into a Green Circle meal, either double the portion of fish or double the portion of brown rice in the Blue Square meal.

Salmon Noodle Salad

- 1 pkg tofu shirataki or plain shirataki noodles
- ½ cup canned salmon, drained and with bones removed

- ¾ cup fat-free or 1% cottage cheese
- your favorite chopped veggies (as much as you want)
- ½ cup cooked or canned chickpeas
- salt and pepper

Prepare shirataki noodles according to package instructions, or simply rinse well with hot water and pat dry. Place them in a big bowl, and toss with salmon, cottage cheese, vegetables, chickpeas, and salt and pepper to taste.

Cheesy Shirataki Alfredo

- 1 pkg fettuccini tofu shirataki noodles
- 2 tbsp low-fat cream cheese or 3 Laughing Cow Light Gourmet Cheese Bites
- ½ cup broccoli florets
- ½ cup zucchini, sliced
- 1 bell pepper, sliced
- salt and pepper
- 2 tbsp grated Parmesan cheese

Prepare shirataki noodles according to package directions, or just rinse them well with hot water, drain, and cut them so they're not quite so long. Pat the noodles dry and place them in a microwave-safe dish along with the cheese. Add broccoli, zucchini, and bell pepper, then sprinkle with salt and pepper to taste and microwave on high for 3 minutes, stirring once at the halfway point. Top the whole thing with Parmesan cheese and serve with a slice of whole grain bread on the side. It's so good! *So good*!

◆ Black Diamond Lunch or Dinner #8

Take-out time! Not in the mood to fuss over dinner? Maybe recovering from a late night followed by a lazy day of skipped exercise and errands (grocery shopping included)? Fear not, my friend; try one of these awesome take-out ideas and keep your waistline in check.

Japanese Take-Out #1

Sushi—yay! Have either 1 order of California rolls, or opt for 2 orders of either cucumber rolls or tuna tekka maki rolls (or a combo of both). Eat them up along with a miso soup and seaweed or green salad.

Japanese Take-Out #2

Sashimi—yay! Have 1 order of tuna or salmon sashimi, 1 order of cucumber or avocado rolls, 1 miso soup, and 1 green salad or seaweed salad.

Japanese Take-Out #3

Have 1 order of salmon or chicken teriyaki, but ask them to skip the rice and give you extra vegetables instead. Eat the yummy teriyaki with a bag of emergency tofu shirataki noodles (which you always have stocked in your fridge now, of course).

Italian Take-Out

Order pasta primavera in tomato sauce (ask for whole wheat noodles if they have them). Eat 1 cup only of the pasta, but feel free to eat any extra tomato sauce or veggies that are in the dish. Just be careful not to have more than 1 cup of noodles. If the portion looks small and your appetite feels large, mix in a bag of shirataki noodles to bulk up the portion size.

BLUE SQUARE• •
Besides the following meal options, be sure to check the Black Diamond meals for Blue Square upgrades.

▓ Blue Square Lunch or Dinner #1
Have any of the Black Diamond lunches or dinners with a serving of fruit on the side.

▓ Blue Square Lunch or Dinner #2
The super-easy frozen entrée meal. Try out these entrees for a quick and scrumptious lunch or dinner idea.

Amy's Kitchen frozen foods
Black Bean Vegetable Enchiladas (eat both); Cheese Lasagna; Tofu Vegetable Lasagna; Thai Stir-Fry; Baked Ziti Bowl; Ravioli Bowl; Cheese Pizza in a Pocket Sandwich; Black Bean or Cheese Enchilada Whole Meal; Country Dinner Whole Meal; Non Dairy Vegetable Pot Pie

Lean Cuisine Spa frozen entrées
Shrimp in a Creamy Seafood Sauce; Butternut Squash Ravioli

PC Blue Menu frozen entrées *(Canada)*
Penne with Roasted Vegetables; Reduced Fat Chicken Lasagna; Rotini with Chicken Pesto

▓ Blue Square Lunch or Dinner #3
Here are some protein- and veggie-packed

restaurant-ordered and home-cooked options that are
sure to keep your taste buds and tummy satisfied.

- McDonald's Grilled Chicken Classic Sandwich with a
  Side Garden Fresh salad or a V8
- Subway Chili with a Veggie Delite Salad dressed with
  any of their light dressings (fat-free Italian and sweet
  onion are good choices)
- McDonald's Southwest Salad with Grilled Chicken
  dressed with 1 packet of Newman's Own Low Fat
  Balsamic Vinaigrette *(US)*
- McDonald's Mighty Caesar Entrée with Warm Grilled
  Chicken dressed with half a packet of Renée's Mighty
  Caesar Light Dressing *(Canada)*
- McDonald's Spicy Thai Chicken Salad with Warm
  Grilled Chicken dressed with half a packet of Renée's
  Asian Sesame Dressing *(Canada)*
- McDonald's Mediterranean Salad with Warm Crispy
  Chicken dressed with 1 packet of Renée's Mediterra-
  nean Greek dressing *(Canada)*

Chicken and Salad

- 1 chicken breast (Tyson brand *(US)* or 200 calories worth of Lilydale Fully Cooked Sliced Chicken
  Breasts (about ⅓ of bag) *(Canada)*, or PC Blue Menu
  Oven Roasted Chicken Breast *(Canada)*)
- mixed greens (as much as you want)
- 4 tbsp cooked chickpeas or edamame
- mixed vegetables of your choice (as much as you'd
  like)
- 3 tbsp (or less) light dressing

Grill the chicken breast (or heat the pre-cooked, sliced chicken breasts). Toss mixed greens with chickpeas or edamame, vegetables, and dressing. Place chicken on salad and serve.

Grilled Chicken with Sweet Potato

- 1 chicken breast (or 200 calories worth of Lilydale Fully Cooked Sliced Chicken Breasts (Tyson brand *(US)*, about ⅓ of bag) *(Canada),* or PC Blue Menu Oven Roasted Chicken Breast *(Canada))*
- 1 small sweet potato
- 1 tsp Gay Lea Light Spreadables *(Canada)* (or Becel Topping and Cooking Spray)
- mixed green salad
- 2 tbsp light dressing (see page 131 for suggestions) or vinaigrette made with 1 tbsp olive oil, 1 tbsp balsamic vinegar, and salt and pepper

Grill the chicken breast (or heat the pre-cooked, sliced chicken breasts). Bake or steam the sweet potato. Top the potato with Light Spreadables or spray with Becel Topping and Cooking Spray. Toss the salad with the dressing and serve on the side.

Halibut with Rice and Vegetables

Have 1 piece of halibut (or your favorite white fish), baked or steamed, with mixed grilled vegetables and ¾ cup brown or basmati rice.

Chicken Quesadilla

- cooking spray
- 2 large La Tortilla Factory Multi Grain Wraps (or any

whole grain tortillas that have approximately
100 calories each)
- ½ cup shredded, part skimmed cheese
- ¼ cup chopped tomatoes or salsa
- ¼ cup light ricotta cheese (I like Allegro 4% milk fat)
- ¼ cup chopped green onion
- salsa
- fat-free sour cream

Heat a skillet over medium heat and spray liberally with
cooking spray. Place 1 tortilla in the skillet to brown.
Sprinkle cheese on the tortilla, then add tomatoes (or
salsa), ricotta, and green onion. Top with a second
tortilla and carefully press down on it with a spatula to
flatten. Flip quesadilla and cook until other side is brown
and cheese is melty. Cut it into triangles and serve with
salsa and fat-free sour cream.

Salmon and Salad
Poach or bake 1 piece of salmon, and serve it with a
salad of mixed greens and vegetables with 1 tablespoon
of sunflower seeds or pumpkin seeds and up to 2 tablespoons of your favorite reduced-calorie salad dressing
(see page 131 for suggestions).

▓ Blue Square Lunch or Dinner #4
If you love noodles and rice, these meals should really
hit the spot. Best of all, the recipes and meal suggestions
are simple and quick to whip together. Enjoy!

Cheesy Spaghetti Squash Dinner
- 1 spaghetti squash

- cooking spray
- ½ cup fat-free cottage cheese or light ricotta cheese
- steamed veggies of your choice

There are two ways to cook spaghetti squash:
1. Preheat oven to 375°F. Cut the squash in half length-wise and scoop out the seeds. (If you microwave the squash for a few minutes first, it's way easier to cut through it.) Line a baking sheet with foil and coat the foil with cooking spray. Place the squash cut side down on the baking sheet and bake for 30 minutes.
2. Alternatively, you can prepare the squash entirely in the microwave. Simply pierce a bunch of holes in it with a fork and microwave it for 20 minutes. When it's done, cut it in half lengthwise and scoop out the seeds.

When the squash is cooked through, use a fork to scoop out the strands. They are delicious, and they really do resemble spaghetti! Top the spaghetti squash with cheese and lots of steamed veggies.

Tuna and Veggie Noodle Salad
So simple, totally filling, and fast!
- 1 pkg tofu shirataki or plain shirataki noodles
- ⅔ cup tuna (about a full can for most brands of tuna), packed in water (drained)
- 1 tbsp olive oil
- 2 tbsp grated Parmesan cheese
- 2-3 tbsp cooked green peas
- salt and pepper

Prepare shirataki noodles according to package directions or simply rinse well under hot water, then rinse them with cold water and pat them dry. Mix noodles with tuna, olive oil, Parmesan cheese, and green peas, and season with salt and pepper to taste.

Feel free to swap the oil and Parm for ¾ cup of low-fat cottage cheese or ricotta cheese instead, and mix in any of your favorite veggies with ½ cup of chickpeas—the variations are endless!

Salmon Cakes

This makes two servings of 3 cakes each. These salmon cakes are fabulous. They make a perfect summer lunch or dinner when served with a bowl of soup and 4 GG Scandinavian Bran Crispbreads topped with fat-free cream cheese and cucumber slices.

- 1 can salmon, drained and with bones removed
- 2 egg whites
- ½ cup rolled oats
- 1 tsp fresh squeezed lemon juice
- ½ cup chopped onion
- 1 tsp fresh ground black pepper
- cooking spray

Preheat oven to 400°F. In a large bowl, mix salmon with egg whites, rolled oats, lemon juice, onion, and pepper. Form into 6 patties. Coat a baking sheet with cooking spray and place the patties on it. Bake them for 10 minutes, flip, and then bake another 10 minutes, until golden.

Japanese Restaurant Order #1

Rolls, soup, salad, and beans—oh my! You can now have 2 orders in total of tuna, salmon, or cucumber tekka maki rolls. Then add 1 miso soup, 1 green or seaweed salad, and 1 order of edamame. If you don't like edamame, feel free to swap them for an order of either salmon or tuna sashimi.

Japanese Restaurant Order #2
Have 1 order (equivalent to 6 average-sized maki rolls) of either Spicy Tuna, Spicy Shrimp, Dragon, Rainbow, or California rolls; 1 miso soup; 1 green or seaweed salad; and either 1 order of edamame or 1 order of tuna or salmon sashimi.

GREEN CIRCLE •
Besides the following meal options, be sure to go back and check the Black Diamond meals for Green Circle upgrades.

● Green Circle Lunch or Dinner #1
Have any of the Black Diamond lunches or dinners with a baked sweet potato.

● Green Circle Lunch or Dinner #2
Have any of the Blue Square lunches or dinners with a serving of fruit.

● Green Circle Lunch or Dinner #3
Hooray for the über-quick frozen entrée! Have any of the following ready-to-go (and delicious—just try them!) meals.

A.C. LaRocco Bruschetta Style Pizza

You can eat the whole thing! And feel free to have a mixed green salad with light vinaigrette on the side. This pizza can be a bit tough to find (I buy mine at Whole Foods), but if you're in the mood for some 'za, this is definitely a treasure worth hunting for. Imagine eating a whole pizza and not feeling guilty for a second! Start hunting, diet rebels.

Amy's Kitchen frozen foods

Try the Mexican Casserole Bowl, the Pesto Tortellini Bowl, the Broccoli Pot Pie, or the Vegetable Pot Pie.

PC Blue Menu frozen entrées *(Canada)*

Have the Reduced Fat Macaroni & 3 Cheeses.

● Green Circle Lunch or Dinner #4

Now your sandwiches can consist of 2 bread servings—yippie! For example, you can choose 2 slices of Food for Life Ezekiel 4:9 Organic Sprouted 100% Whole Grain Flourless Bread, 2 slices of Dimpflmeier Pumpernickel Bread *(Canada)*, 1 Weight Watchers Bagel, or 4 slices of Weight Watchers 100% Whole Wheat Sliced Bread. It's totally up to you. (To remind yourself of all the bread options, flip back to page 107). Try some of these awesome sandwich ideas, and pair them up with any one of the 100-calorie soup ideas listed on page 128 (or make your own).

- 1 slice light havarti cheese, melted, with sliced tomatoes and fresh basil
- 2 tablespoons of light cream cheese, 3 slices lox or smoked salmon (about 100 grams or 3 ounces),

cucumber slices, tomato slices, thinly sliced red onion, and capers to taste
- 3 tablespoons of hummus, 1 tablespoon of toasted
pine nuts, cucumber slices, tomato slices, and alfalfa
sprouts (if you have time, grilled eggplant also works
well)

Guacamole

- 1 ripe avocado
- juice of half a lime
- pinch of chili flakes (or to taste)
- salt and pepper

For an awesome guac in minutes, mash up the avocado
and mix in the lime juice and chili flakes. Add salt and
pepper to taste.

Pair 2 tablespoons of guacamole with 4 slices of turkey and half a sliced apple. This is such a good sandwich
idea, I just made one for myself this very instant!

● Green Circle Lunch or Dinner #5

Full, rich meals—what a concept! Here are some awesome
ideas that are great for your waistline and your palate.
Many of these meal ideas can be found at restaurants, or
you can make them at home. Seriously, people; they're
super-easy. Even if you're more of a ball-busta' than a bala-
busta (look it up), you can still succeed with these.
- Buy a rotisserie chicken at the supermarket. Eat an
amount equivalent to 1 breast (save the rest for left-
overs)—white meat only, without skin. Serve it with
½ cup of cooked brown rice and unlimited steamed
green beans sprayed with Becel Topping and Cooking

Spray and topped with 1 or 2 tablespoons of toasted
slivered almonds.

- Order a Swiss Chalet quarter chicken breast or leg
  dinner *(Canada)*. This dinner includes a chicken
  breast or leg without skin, rotisserie vegetables, green
  salad, and roll.
- Crispy Chicken Breasts with Roasted Butternut
  Squash, served alongside a green salad with light
  vinaigrette:

Crispy Chicken Breasts
This makes two servings.

- 10 Multifibre Melba Toast rounds
- 2 tsp flax seeds
- seasoning salt
- cooking spray
- ¼ cup egg whites
- ¼ cup skim milk
- 2 chicken breasts
- 2 tsp Becel Light or Gay Lea Light Spreadables
  (Canada)

Preheat oven to 425°F. To make breading, put Melba
Toast, flax seeds, and seasoning salt to taste in a plastic
bag. Mash it with a rolling pin until the cracker mixture
is all crumbly.

Coat a baking sheet with cooking spray. Beat egg
whites and skim milk, and pour into a shallow bowl. Dip
the chicken breasts in the egg wash, then coat them with
the breading. Lay them on the cookie sheet. Melt Becel
Light or Gay Lea Light Spreadables in the microwave,
and then lightly drizzle one teaspoon on each chicken

breast. Bake for 20 minutes, or until the chicken is cooked through and the breading is golden.

Roasted Butternut Squash
One serving of squash is about 1 cup cooked.
- pre-peeled, diced squash (it comes prepackaged in most produce sections)
- 1 tbsp olive oil
- cooking spray
- kosher salt

Preheat oven to 425°F. In a bowl, toss the squash with olive oil until well coated. Coat a baking sheet with cooking spray and place the squash on it. Sprinkle a few pinches of kosher salt on the squash. Bake for 40 minutes, or until the squash gets crispy, like fries. YUM. You can also add fresh rosemary for a nice flavor.

Chicken Tenders with Steamed Zucchini and Potato Skins

Chicken Tenders
This makes four servings.
- 450 g (1 lb) boneless, skinless chicken breasts, cut into strips
- ½ cup buttermilk
- cooking spray
- ½ cup grated Parmesan cheese
- ½ cup Italian-style whole wheat breadcrumbs (I use Edward and Sons)

Marinate the chicken strips in buttermilk for 30 minutes. Preheat the oven to 500°F. Coat a baking sheet with
cooking spray.

Combine Parmesan cheese and breadcrumbs in a
shallow dish. Dredge the chicken strips in the bread-
crumb/cheese mixture, then lay them on the prepared
baking sheet. Bake for approximately 12 to 15 minutes,
until chicken is cooked through.

Steamed Zucchini

This makes four servings.
- 4 medium zucchini
- 1 tbsp olive oil
- 1 tbsp grated Parmesan cheese
- salt and pepper

Cut the zucchini in half crosswise, then into quarters
lengthwise. Steam the zucchini until they are softened
but not mushy. Lightly drizzle the zucchini with oil and
sprinkle with Parmesan cheese and salt and pepper to
taste.

Potato Skins

This makes one serving.
- 1 large baking potato
- salsa (unlimited)
- 2 tbsp fat-free sour cream
- green onions (unlimited)

Poke several holes in the potato using a fork. Wrap the
potato in a paper towel, and cook it in the microwave on
high for 7 minutes. When it's cooled a bit, cut it in half

and scoop out most of the potato so you are left with the skins and just a small amount of the potato inside. Spoon salsa, fat-free sour cream, and green onions into the skins. Both halves make for one serving.

- Grill a chicken breast, or heat up ⅓ bag of Lilydale or PC Blue Menu cooked, sliced chicken breasts *(Canada))*; steam 1 small baked sweet potato and top it with 1 teaspoon Gay Lea Light Spreadables *(Canada)* or Becel Topping and Cooking spray; and serve with mixed greens tossed with light vinaigrette dressing.
- Baked Fish with Roasted Cauliflower (served with a baked or steamed sweet potato or ¾ cup brown rice or quinoa):

Baked Fish

- cooking spray
- 1 piece of white fish, such as tilapia or halibut
- ¼ cup chopped bell pepper
- ¼ cup sliced mushrooms
- ¼ cup sliced onion
- 1 tbsp water or chicken broth
- salt and pepper
- ¼ cup salsa
- 2 tbsp grated Parmesan cheese

Spray a microwave-safe dish with cooking spray. Place the fish in the dish along with the vegetables. Add in water or chicken broth and salt and pepper. Microwave on high, covered but with a small opening for steam to escape, for 5 minutes, until the fish is cooked through and the vegetables are tender. When done, drain off some of the liquid. Add salsa on top of the veggies and cook for 1 more minute. Top with Parmesan cheese.

Roasted Cauliflower

- 1 cauliflower head
- 1–2 tbsp olive oil
- Kosher salt

Preheat oven to 400°F. On a cookie sheet, break the cauliflower into small florets. Sprinkle the olive oil on the cauliflower and toss to coat. Season with kosher salt and bake for 25 minutes, or until brown.

- Have 1 piece of poached or baked salmon with ½ cup of brown rice and a salad of mixed greens and vegetables topped with 1 tablespoon of sunflower seeds or pumpkin seeds and a light dressing.
- Have a 6 oz filet mignon (lean) with steamed vegetables and half a baked white potato or sweet potato.
- Chicken Fajitas and Kale Chips

Chicken Fajitas

This recipe makes two servings.

- 225 g (½ lb) boneless, skinless chicken breasts cut into thin strips
- 1 tsp canola oil
- ½ onion, sliced
- 1 bell pepper, sliced into strips
- 2 garlic cloves, finely chopped
- 1 tbsp chili powder
- 1 ½ tsp ground cumin
- 1 tsp red pepper flakes
- salt and pepper
- 2 large multigrain tortillas (La Tortilla Factory Multi Grain Wraps are best)

- salsa (unlimited)
- 2 tbsp fat-free sour cream
- shredded lettuce (unlimited)
- 6 tbsp shredded light cheese

In a large wok, heat the oil to medium high and cook the chicken until nearly done. Add the vegetables and seasonings, and mix well. Cover and cook until the peppers are tender and the vegetables are starting to brown. Warm up the tortillas according to package directions. Dress the fajitas with the chicken and vegetables, as well as salsa, fat-free sour cream, shredded lettuce, and shredded cheese.

Kale Chips

These are amazing!
- 1 bunch kale
- 1 tbsp olive oil
- 1 tsp kosher salt
- cooking spray
- apple cider vinegar (optional)

Preheat the oven to 375°F. Simply tear the leaves of one bunch of kale into bite-size pieces. Pour olive oil into a large mixing bowl, then toss in the kale leaves and mix well until coated. Throw in the salt and mix some more. Coat a baking sheet with cooking spray, and place the kale on the baking sheet. Bake for 20 minutes, but don't bake for any longer because they're quick to burn. Add apple cider vinegar to taste for salt and vinegar chips, if you like.

● Green Circle Lunch or Dinner #6

These ideas below really highlight the fact that eating for health and weight loss doesn't have to be synonymous with labor-intensive cooking and unsatisfying foods. Despite what you may have been duped into believing before, if it tastes good, it won't necessarily wreak havoc on your diet. Just sample some of these meal suggestions, recipes, and take-out ideas if you're not convinced. You'll be a converted rebel in no time!

Pasta Primavera

Combine 1 ½ cups cooked Dreamfields pasta (or 1 cup cooked whole wheat pasta) with a tomato-based primavera sauce topped with 2 tablespoons of grated Parmesan cheese. Have a green salad with a light vinaigrette on the side.

Pesto Pasta

- ⅓ cup walnuts
- 1 tbsp olive oil
- 1 bunch fresh basil leave (about ½ cup)
- kosher salt and fresh ground pepper
- 1 cup cooked Dreamfields pasta; or ½ cup cooked whole wheat pasta combined with 1 bag prepared plain or tofu shirataki noodles to expand the portion size
- 2 tbsp grated Parmesan cheese

To make pesto sauce, preheat the oven to 400°F. Toast the walnuts on a baking sheet in the oven for a few minutes (watch closely so they don't burn). Put the toasted walnuts in a blender along with the olive oil, basil, and salt and pepper to paste. Pulse until combined. Add a bit of warm water to thin the pesto to a desired consistency, and pulse again.

You can use the entire pesto sauce as one serving, but it's a rich sauce, so to save calories, use less if you don't need all of it to coat the pasta. Top your pasta with Parmesan cheese and serve with a green salad and low-calorie dressing.

Mediterranean Take-Out

Order 1 skewer of chicken, 1 mixed green salad (ask for the dressing on the side), and 1 pita (whole wheat, if they have it) with 2 tablespoons of hummus on the side.

Greek Take-Out

Order 1 skewer of chicken souvlaki, 1 side Greek salad without dressing (just use balsamic vinegar to dress), and ½ pita bread (about 4 triangles) with up to 2 table-spoons of tzatziki dip.

Vietnamese Take-Out

Get 1 order of chicken Pho (a Vietnamese noodle soup made with chicken broth and pieces of chicken). Eat up the whole thing, noodles and all, and heck, you can even have one spring roll on the side.

Thai Take-Out

Order either a lemongrass- or hot-and-sour-based soup with either chicken or shrimp, and have one order of fresh salad rolls on the side. (Salad rolls are not deep fried. They're wrapped in rice paper, and you can often get either vegetarian, shrimp, or chicken varieties.)

CHAPTER 15

REBEL-ICIOUS SNACKS

Who doesn't love snacking? You can—and should—have one, two, or even three snacks throughout the day along with your meals. I often suggest having one snack in the mid-afternoon and one in the evening; if you have a morning workout, you can add another snack mid-morning. So here I've given you some of my favorite snack suggestions. And I've organized them the only real logical way: by craving.

Many of the snacks I've listed here give ranges of amounts, so if you're attempting more of a Black Diamond Rebel Diet, stick with the lower end of the range. If you're a Green Circle kind of gal, go ahead and indulge in the upper end of the range. Also, some of the snacks are less indulgent, but still delicious and super-healthy (such as two tangerines), while some are more indulgent but still totally Rebel Diet–acceptable (like a small Dairy Queen strawberry sundae). So make sure you mix and match to take full advantage of all the wonderful options open to you.

One last thing: be sure to make your way to the very end of the snack list, 'cause that's where I list "free" snacks. You can have as many of these as you like!

Okay, truly last thing: many of the Black Diamond or Blue Square breakfasts make awesome snacks as well.

FRUITY •

- 2 tangerines
- 1 ½ cups fresh or frozen grapes (about 25)
- 1 ½ cups blueberries, raspberries, or strawberries in 1 to 2 tablespoons of cream, milk, or light coconut milk *You can also wash fresh berries, sprinkle sweetener on them, and then freeze them. They taste great frozen and take longer to eat, so they're great to snack on.*
- 1 cup of diced watermelon
- 1 cup of cherries
- 1 bag of Sensible Foods Crunch Dried Fruit or a couple handfuls of Bare Fruit Granny Smith Apple Chips
- 3 prunes or figs along with 10 almonds
- ½ to 1 cup of unsweetened applesauce sprinkled with cinnamon, with or without sweetener
- 1 Breyers 100 Calorie Ice Cream Cup with ½ cup of blueberries on top
- McDonald's Fruit 'n Yogurt Parfait
- McDonald's Blueberry Raspberry Sundae *(Canada)* or Strawberry Sundae

CHEESY •

- 2 to 4 Laughing Cow Light Gourmet Cheese Bites along with a sliced pear
- 2 Mini Babybel Light Cheese snacks
- Celery sticks topped with 2 tablespoons of Cheez Whiz Light and 1 tablespoon of raisins (your mom called these "Ants on a Log")
- Broccoli or cauliflower florets dipped into 2 tablespoons of Cheez Whiz Light
- Melt it in the microwave as per the directions on the jar to make it a warm dip.

Warm Broccoli Slaw

- ½ bag broccoli slaw
- 2 tbsp Cheez Whiz Light
- salt and pepper

Empty the broccoli slaw into a microwave-safe dish and spoon the Cheez Whiz Light on top. Microwave on high for 1 minute. Add salt and pepper to taste, and you've got a healthy high-fiber, low-cal version of macaroni and cheese—if you really stretch your imagination!

- 30 grams (1 ounce) of your favorite cheese, preferably light or part skim, with a glass of red wine
- 2 to 4 thick, high-fiber crackers such as GG Scandinavian Bran Crispbreads, Wasa Light Crispbreads, or Ryvita Light Rye Crispbreads, with 2 Laughing Cow Light Gourmet Cheese Bites melted on top. Place the cheese on the crackers and put the crackers in the microwave on high for 20 seconds. Once done, add tomato or cucumbers on top if you like.

CREAMY ·································

- 1 to 2 snack-size containers (about ¼ to ½ cup) of low-fat (2% or less) cottage cheese, mixed with 1 to 2 snack-size containers of low-calorie fruit yogurt. *I mix Breakstone's cottage cheese with Yoplait Source 0% Raspberry Yogurt.*
- ½ banana with ½ cup of low-fat cottage cheese, 1 tablespoon of slivered almonds, and cinnamon and sweetener to taste. *You can either eat this cold or warm it up in the microwave for 30 seconds or so.*
- 2 to 4 thick, high-fiber crackers with 2 tablespoons of

low-fat cream cheese, some cucumber slices, and salt
and pepper to taste
- 2 to 4 thick, high-fiber crackers with 2 tablespoons of
Guiltless Gourmet Fat Free Black Bean Dip, 2 tablespoons of fat free sour cream, and 2 tablespoons of salsa
- ½ to 1 cup baby carrots dipped into 2 tablespoons of
light ranch dressing
- ½ bell pepper sliced and dipped into 3 tablespoons of
light hummus
- 1 medium skim milk latte

NUTTY •
- 1 to 2 handfuls (about 10 to 20) of almonds, walnuts,
or pistachios
- 5 to 10 brazil nuts

Peanut Butter Cracker-Sandwiches
Make peanut butter "sandwiches" by spreading 1 tablespoon of light peanut butter or natural nut butter on
3 Kavli Crispy Thin Crispbreads or 4 Multigrain Melba
Toast rounds, then place 3 or 4 more crackers on top to
make your peanut butter cracker-sandwiches. Feel free
to add low-calorie jam or unsweetened applesauce along
with the peanut butter.

- 2 tablespoons of prepared PB2 spread or 1 tablespoon of
natural nut butter on a toasted Weight Watchers Bagel
- 1 large glass of unsweetened vanilla or chocolate almond milk with a sliced apple dipped in 1 tablespoon
of light peanut butter
- Celery sticks (as many as you want!) with 1 tablespoon of light peanut butter or 2 tablespoons of
prepared PB2 spread

WARM ·

- 1 cup of Imagine Organic soup or 1 Campbell's Soup at Hand
- ½ baked sweet potato with unsweetened applesauce on top
- 40 edamame beans (about ½ cup shelled beans)
- 1 packet of multigrain oatmeal made with boiling water, sprinkled with cinnamon and sweetener to taste and topped with ½ cup of unsweetened applesauce and 1 tablespoon of slivered almonds

SWEET· ·

- 1 Carnation Hot Chocolate Light packet dissolved in ¾ cup of boiling water; you can add ¼ cup of skim milk and 1 dollop of light whipped cream as well
- 1 Breyers 100 Calorie Ice Cream Cup
- 1 Skinny Cow Ice Cream Sandwich (vanilla or chocolate)
- 1 Skinny Cow Ice Cream Cone
- 20 Miss Meringue mini sugar-free meringues
- A 100 calorie snack-size bag of popcorn (such as Orville Redenbacher's 100 Calorie Mini Bags or PC Blue Menu 100 Calorie Mini Bags *(Canada))* sprayed with Becel Topping and Cooking Spray. *You can also sprinkle cinnamon sweetener on top. Make cinnamon sweetener by mixing cinnamon and your preferred sweetener to taste.*
- A 100 calorie snack-size bag of popcorn combined with 1 bag of Sensible Foods Crunch Dried Fruit
- YummyEarth candy (6 Organic Candy Drops or 4 Organic Lollipops)
- 1 No Pudge! Fat Free Fudge Brownie

- 1 cup of Nature's Path Kamut Puffs in ½ cup of skim or unsweetened almond milk, sweetened with cinnamon sweetener.
  Feel free to add 1 bag of Sensible Foods Crunch Dried Fruit.
- 1 Doctor's CarbRite Diet Bar (any flavor)
- 1 FullBar (any flavor)
- 1 Chocolite Protein Bar (any flavor)
- 2 New Sun cookies
- 1 Vitalicious 100 calorie Vitatop.
  This is great warmed up and topped with a dollop of light whipped cream.
- 1 President's Choice Imported Meringue Nest filled with ½ cup of berries and 1 or 2 dollops of light whipped cream
- 1 Häagen-Dazs 97% Fat Free Sorbet and Yogourt bar (with fewer than 100 calories!)
- 1 snack-size container (about ⅓ cup) of low-fat (2% or less) cottage cheese with ½ teaspoon of vanilla extract and 1 packet of sweetener mixed in.
  Instead of cottage cheese, you can have ⅓ cup of light ricotta cheese, and you can mix in 1 snack-size low-cal Jell-O dessert instead of the vanilla and sweetener—it works really well!
- 1 McDonald's Ice Cream Cone (chocolate or vanilla)
- 1 Wendy's Junior Frosty
- 1 small Dairy Queen chocolate or vanilla soft-serve cone (in a regular cone, not a sugar cone or waffle cone)
- 1 small Dairy Queen strawberry sundae
- ½ small Dairy Queen Oreo Blizzard
  Now, this is a real treat, but you can have it and still totally be on track with your skinni-mizing,

shrink-a-cizing Rebel Diet mission so long as you only eat half. Split one with your best friend and savor every spoonful!

Orange Pineapple Jell-O Dessert

- 1 packet low-calorie orange Jell-O gelatin
- ¾ cup boiling water
- 1 cup club soda, cold
- ½ cup canned mandarin orange segments, drained
- 1 cup canned pineapple chunks, drained (do not use fresh pineapple)
- light whipped cream (optional)

In a medium-sized bowl, dissolve the Jell-O in the boiling water. Stir until completely dissolved. Refrigerate for 15 minutes, then stir in club soda and refrigerate for another 30 minutes, until slightly thickened. Add mandarin orange segments and pineapple chunks; stir gently. Refrigerate for another 3 to 4 hours, until firm. Top with light whipped cream, if you wish. And feel free to eat the whole dish, as it only has about 100 calories!

Pumpkin Cheesecake Dessert

- ¼ cup light ricotta cheese
- ¼ cup canned pumpkin or butternut squash baby food
- sweetener, cinnamon, and nutmeg
- a few graham crackers

In a small bowl, mix ricotta and pumpkin or butternut squash, and add sweetener, cinnamon, and nutmeg to taste. Stir to combine. Crumble graham crackers on top.

FREE STUFF! •

If you're feeling like munching on something in addition to your meals and snacks, grab one of these fab free foods at anytime. Also, feel free to add any of these to your meals.

- White, green, yellow, and red vegetables (think lettuce greens, mushrooms, onions, garlic, cucumbers, pickles, bell peppers, hearts of palm, celery, zucchini, tomatoes, broccoli, cauliflower, etc.), either raw or lightly steamed
- Vegetable cocktail, such as V8, or a virgin Bloody Caesar
- Water or soda water
- Black, green, or white tea
- Black coffee (but no more than 2 to 3 cups per day)
- Vegetable broths or veggie soups, such as homemade cabbage soup, consommé or stock made just with vegetables, single-serving soup cups with 60 calories or fewer, and miso soup packets
- Low-cal gelatin desserts (FYI: Haddar brand is made with Splenda, Jell-O brand is made with aspartame)
- Diet Snapple on Ice Pops
- Sugar-free gum

CHAPTER 16
F&*% DIETING!

So you did it! You're now a Rebel Diet expert, armed with loads of meal and snack ideas to help you face each obstacle, craving, and hunger pang that comes your merry way. Remember, on the Rebel Diet, you can have frozen foods, take-out meals, sweets, fast food, and easy home-cooked food. And you will reach your goal, looking better and feeling healthier than you even imagined possible once you get there—I promise! But just in case you need a little hand holding before you begin, I have sketched out what some sample days could look like on this plan. I have purposely selected difficult days—days when you may be exhausted, or driving from meeting to meeting, or dealing with major PMS-style mood swings—because if you can cope on those days, you can lose weight any day.

Each sample day includes three meals and two snacks. For each of the three meals, I've given you Black Diamond, Blue Square, and Green Circle options so you can select the one that best suits you. (Except for the final meal plan; when you have a killer workout, you deserve all Green Circle meals!) If you don't like any of the meals or snacks, just flip back to the earlier chapters in Part Three and choose any meal you like instead. And don't forget, you can add "free" foods in any time you want. Hop back on the weight-loss wagon, ladies, and relax. This time there's no reason to fall off!

I'M TOO TIRED TO DO ANY REAL COOKING
TODAY •

Breakfast

◆ 1 cup of Nature's Path Kamut Puffs cereal with ½ cup skim milk or unsweetened almond milk; add cinnamon sweetener to taste

■ 1 apple with 1 slice of light havarti cheese, 1 Mini Babybel Light Cheese, or 30 grams (1 ounce) of cheddar cheese

● 2 Van's 97% Fat Free Waffles with either half a sliced banana or ¾ cup berries on top; add Walden Farms Calorie Free Pancake Syrup (or your favorite calorie-free or light pancake syrup)

Lunch

◆ McDonald's Grilled Chicken Snack Wrap *(US) with* Grilled Caesar Chicken Snack Wrap *(Canada)* or Ranch with a V8 or side salad

■ 1 large Subway salad with turkey, ham, tuna, or grilled chicken, with or without cheese, using sweet onion, honey mustard, or fat-free Italian dressing to dress. What the heck—add a bag of Baked Lay's chips on the side as well!

● Have a Blue Square frozen entrée (choose either a PC Blue Menu, Amy's Kitchen, or Lean Cuisine Spa meal from the Blue Square list on page 125) and pair it with a serving of fruit, or choose a Green Circle frozen entrée, such as Amy's Mexican Casserole Bowl.

Dinner

◆ Japanese Take-Out: Have 1 order of either chicken or salmon teriyaki dinner, but ask them to skip the rice and to give you extra vegetables instead. Then, grab a bag of shirataki noodles from your fridge and combine the noodles with the teriyaki meal. Yum!

■ Japanese Take-Out: Have 1 order (equivalent to 6 average-sized maki rolls) of either Spicy Tuna, Spicy Shrimp, Dragon, Rainbow, or California rolls; 1 miso soup; 1 green or seaweed salad; and either 1 small order of edamame or one order of tuna or salmon sashimi.

● Greek Take-Out: Have 1 skewer chicken souvlaki; 1 side Greek salad without dressing (just use balsamic vinegar to dress); and ½ pita bread (about 4 triangles) with up to 2 tablespoons of tzatziki dip.

Snacks

1. 1 Skinny Cow Ice Cream Sandwich
2. 1 grapefruit topped with cinnamon sweetener to taste

ROAD TRIP! NO MORE DRIVE-THRU DISASTERS •••••••••••••••••••••••••••

Breakfast

◆ 1 Vitalicious 100 Calorie VitaTop

■ 2 New Sun Cookies, Apple Cinnamon flavor

● 1 McDonald's Breakfast Burrito

Lunch

◆ Clif 20g Protein Builder's Bar along with 1 cup unsweetened almond milk or a V8

▨ Wendy's Hot Stuffed Baked Potato personalized to include any or all of the following toppings: chives, broccoli, 3 ounces of chili, or a dollop of sour cream

● Subway 6 inch sub: Have a turkey, ham, or veggie delite sub with unlimited veggies and up to 2 slices of cheese; have it with either a soup of the day (as long as it's not cream-based) or a bag of Baked Lay's potato chips

Dinner

◆ McDonald's Bacon Ranch Salad with Grilled Chicken dressed with 1 packet of Newman's Own Low Fat Balsamic Dressing *(US)* or McDonald's Spicy Thai Chicken Salad with Warm Grilled Chicken dressed with 1 packet of Renée's Ravin' Raspberry Dressing *(Canada)*

▨ McDonald's Grilled Chicken Classic Sandwich with a Side Garden Fresh Salad or a V8

● 2 Tim Hortons Chicken Wrap Snackers (either Barbecue Chicken, Chicken Salad, or Chicken Ranch) and a side soup of the day

Snacks

1. 1 McDonald's Fruit 'n Yogurt Parfait
2. 10 to 20 almonds

HELP—I FEEL LIKE MUNCHING! • • • • • • • • • • • •

Breakfast

◆ ¾ cup low-fat cottage cheese with 1 to 2 tablespoons of Multi-Grain Cheerios (add cinnamon sweetener, if you like)

■ ½ cup Astro Original Balkan Style Yogourt or 1 cup of fat-free plain yogurt with 1 bag Sensible Foods Crunch Dried Fruit mixed in

● Egg White and Yolk Omelet (recipe on page 160) with 1 serving of crunchy crackers (5 Kavli Crispy Thin Crispbreads, 5 Multifibre Melba Toast rounds, 4 GG Scandinavian Bran Crispbreads, 4 Wasa Light Crispbreads, 4 Ryvita Light Rye Crispbreads, or 1 sheet whole wheat matzo) topped with 2 tablespoons of Cheez Whiz Light

Lunch

◆ Bean and Seed Salad (recipe on page 180)

■ Cobb Salad topped with 113 grams (4 ounces) lean deli meat (recipe on page 180)

● Pasta Salad using the full cup of penne and 3 tablespoons of cooked chickpeas (recipe on page 183)

Dinner

◆ 1 bowl of "Creamy" Protein-Packed Tomato Soup with crumbled crackers (recipe on page 173)

■ Chicken Quesadilla (recipe on page 190)

● Chicken Fajitas and Kale Chips (recipes on page 201-202)

Snacks
1. Orville Redenbacher's 100 Calorie Mini Bag of popcorn mixed with a handful of Bare Fruit Granny Smith Apple Chips
2. Carrot and celery sticks dipped in 2 tablespoons of light ranch dressing

I NEED BREAD, SO SUE ME • • • • • • • • • • • • • • • • •

Breakfast
◆ 2 slices of Weight Watchers 100% Whole Wheat Sliced Bread topped with 2 tablespoons of Cheez Whiz Light and sliced tomatoes

■ 3 slices of French Toast (recipe on page 163)

● Egg White Omelet (recipe on page 160) with tomato slices, 3 slices of low-fat chicken, turkey, or ham bacon, and 1 bread serving, such as 1 slice of toasted Ezekiel 4:9 Sprouted Whole Grain Bread

Lunch
◆ Amy's Bean & Cheese Burrito (you can substitute any of the other Black Diamond Amy's Kitchen suggestions from page 125, such as the Teriyaki Wrap or Spinach Pizza in a Pocket Sandwich if you like)

■ 1 Homemade Chicken Wrap with 3 tablespoons of shredded part skim cheese (recipe on page 175)

● 2 tablespoons of Guacamole (recipe on page 196) with 4 slices of turkey and half a sliced apple on 2 servings of bread, paired with a 100 calorie serving of your favorite soup (see suggestions on page 128)

Dinner

Cheesy Shirataki Alfredo with a slice of whole grain ◆ bread on the side (recipe on page 186)

■ Stuffed Greek Pita using ¾ of the pita (see page 176 for recipe)

● Mediterranean Take-Out: Order 1 skewer of chicken, 1 mixed green salad (ask for the dressing on the side), and 1 pita (whole wheat if they have it) with 2 tablespoons of hummus on the side

Snacks

1. 1 ½ cups frozen grapes
2. Celery sticks topped with 2 tablespoons of Cheez Whiz Light and 1 tablespoon of raisins

I'M HAVING A ROUGH DAY AND I JUST WANT TO BE A KID AGAIN. COMFORT ME! • • • • • • • • • • • •

Breakfast

◆ 1 bread serving toasted and topped with a light coating of Becel Topping and Cooking Spray and sprinkled with cinnamon sweetener

■ 1 Amy's Apple Toaster Pop or Strawberry Toaster Pop

● 2 Nature's Path Frozen Waffles with Walden Farms Calorie Free Pancake Syrup, with a grapefruit on the side sprinkled with cinnamon sweetener

Lunch
◆ Make a delicious sandwich using 2 bread servings (such as 2 slices of Ezekiel 4:9 Sprouted Whole Grain Bread), 1 tablespoon of light peanut butter, 1 tablespoon of Walden Farms Calorie Free Apple Butter, and half a sliced apple or banana

■ Amy's Cheese Pizza in a Pocket Sandwich

● PC Blue Menu Reduced Fat Macaroni & 3 Cheeses

Dinner
◆ Lean Cuisine Spa Creamy Chicken Alfredo entrée

■ Cheesy Spaghetti Squash Dinner (recipe on page 191)

● Chicken Tenders with Steamed Zucchini and Potato Skins (recipes on page 198)

Snacks
1. Two Mini Babybel Light Cheeses
2. ½ small Dairy Queen Oreo Blizzard

I HAVE SERIOUS PMS—HELP ME! • • • • • • • • • • •

Breakfast
◆ 2 slices Weight Watchers 100% Whole Wheat Sliced Bread topped either with 1 tablespoon prepared chocolate PB2 spread or with Becel Topping and Cooking Spray and cinnamon sweetener

▮ 1 Doctor's CarbRite Diet Bar, S'mores flavor, (or a 200 calorie BALANCE Bar), with a cup of unsweetened vanilla almond milk

● Iced Mocha (recipe on page 162) with 1 Vitalicious 100 Calorie VitaTop

Lunch
◆ 1 Chocolate Banana Smoothie (recipe on page 166)

▮ 1 large Subway salad (with either chicken, tuna salad, turkey, or ham, and either fat-free Italian or sweet onion dressing) with a bag of Baked Lay's chips on the side

● Egg Salad Sandwich (recipe on page 172) using 2 whole eggs, 4 egg whites, and 2 bread servings

Dinner
◆ Japanese Take-Out: 1 order of tuna or salmon sashimi, 1 order of cucumber or avocado rolls, 1 miso soup, and 1 seaweed or green salad

■ Here's a good, clean meal if you're bloated: 1 piece baked or steamed halibut (or your favorite white fish) served with mixed grilled vegetables and ¾ cup cooked brown or basmati rice

● 1 A.C. LaRocco Bruschetta Style Pizza (you can eat the whole thing!)

Snacks

1. 1 small Dairy Queen chocolate soft-serve cone
2. 1 No Pudge! Fat Free Fudge Brownie

I WORKED OUT HARD AND I'M HUNGRY TODAY (SO I'M EATING ALL GREEN CIRCLES!) • • • • • • • •

Breakfast

● PC Blue Menu Steel-Cut Oats with Wild Blueberries along with 4 slices Canadian back bacon

● Egg White and Yolk Omelet (recipe on page 160) served with 1 slice of Ezekiel 4:9 Sprouted Whole Grain Bread, toasted and topped with Walden Farms Calorie Free Apple Butter

● Clif 20g Protein Builder's Bar and 1 cup of unsweetened almond milk

Lunch

● 1 Havarti, Tomato, and Basil Sandwich (see page 195 for recipe)

● 1 Weight Watchers Bagel with 2 tablespoons of light cream cheese, 3 slices of smoked salmon or lox (about

100 grams or 3 ounces), cucumber slices, tomato slices, and sliced red onion and capers to taste

● Subway Chili: Have a bowl of chili along with a Veggie Delite Salad with any of their light dressings (fat-free Italian and sweet onion are good choices). You can have a bag of Baked Lay's chips or an apple on the side.

Dinner
● Pesto Pasta (see page 203 for recipe)

● Buy a rotisserie chicken, and have an amount equivalent to 1 breast—white meat only, without skin. Serve it with ½ cup of cooked brown rice and unlimited steamed green beans sprayed with Becel Topping and Cooking Spray and topped with 1 or 2 tablespoons of toasted slivered almonds.

● Have a 6 ounce filet mignon with unlimited steamed vegetables and half a baked sweet potato.

Snacks
1. Chocolate Banana Protein Shake (recipe on page 166)
2. 1 Breyers 100 Calorie Ice Cream Cup with ½ cup berries

Okay, rebel darlings, we've covered everything you need to know about breaking the dreadful "diet" rules, you're up to date on the best new foods on the market (and they're now in your pantry), and your head is full of hundreds of awesome new ideas for meals and snacks. There's nothing to stop you now, you have no more excuses, and you're ready to start skiing the rebel diet slopes…or shall I say ski-nny-ing your way through the Black Diamond, Blue Square, and Green Circle meals!

You're going to eat; you're going to cheat (actually, you'll just feel like you're cheating while enjoying your Dairy Queen Blizzard, but you and I know you're not cheating at all!); and best of all, you're going to defeat your weight-loss struggles once and for all. Let's all shout it loud and clear for everybody to hear: Eat. Cheat. Defeat. Fuck old-school dieting FOREVER!

ACKNOWLEDGMENTS

Thank you to my agent, Rick Broadhead, who introduced me to Leah Fairbank, my awesome, enthusiastic editor, and Jennifer Smith, the publisher who allowed this all to happen. Thank you to Jenny Govier for her amazing edits and comments—the book would not be what is today without the dizzying red underlines and notes. And to the rest of the team at Wiley: thank you for your dedication, creativity, and hard work. To my family, friends, colleagues and clients, thank you for your feedback and for listening patiently as I excitedly blabbed on and on. And last but not least, thanks to Ty for being my brutally honest recipe and product guinea pig and for finally admitting that I can cook!

ABOUT THE AUTHOR

Melissa Hershberg, MD, is a medical doctor who provides comprehensive family practice, preventive health services, and weight loss expertise at The Toronto Clinic™, a pioneering integrative health care facility. Originally from Winnipeg, Dr. Hershberg completed her undergraduate degree on scholarship at McGill University and subsequently obtained her family medicine degree at the University of Toronto. She is the author of the top selling book *The Hershberg Diet*, and is medical director for U Weight Loss® chains across Canada.

Dr. Hershberg's experiences in competitive gymnastics and fitness coupled with her training in science and medicine have afforded her with a unique and highly respected knowledge base. In addition to practicing medicine, she is a freelance writer, dynamic public speaker and recurring correspondent for CTV news. To learn more about Dr. Hershberg or to book a consultation with her, visit www.melissahershberg.com.

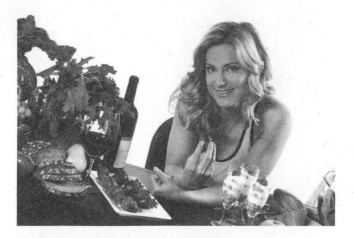

INDEX

See also Recipes and
Product indexes, below.

A
abdominal circumference,
97, 99
abstinence, 13
adenosine receptor
antagonist, 92
adenosine triphosphate
(ATP), 44, 45
alcohol, 81–87
almond, 115
butter, 136
extract, 137
milk, 19, 116–117
antioxidants, 89, 90, 96
appetizers, frozen, 125–126
apples, 114–115
applesauce, 137
arteries, and fat, 60
artificial sweeteners, 41

B
bacon, 111–112, 138
bagels, 51, 109
baggy clothing, 102
bake-dried fruits, 21, 141
bakery, 107–109, 131
balsamic vinegar, 134
bar shot, 82
basmati rice, 52
beans, 54–55
beer, 82–84
beverages, 123–124
Big Mac, 19, 69, 75
big meals, 78–79

Black Diamond, explained,
148
black tea, 90, 91
blender drinks, 83
bloating, 29–30, 31, 55, 109
blood sugar, 47
Blue Square, explained, 148
Body Mass Index (BMI),
98–100
body shape, 99
body shapers, 102
booze, 81
"botox clock," 10
bran cereals, 130–131
bread, 50–51, 107–109
breadcrumbs, 109
breakfast, 35
and calorie ladder, 78
foods, frozen, 127
meats, 111–112
menus, 151–167
brown fat, 61
brownie mix, 142
brown rice, 52, 139
bulk food, 115–116
butter, 118
buttermilk, 117

C
caffeine, 92
calorie ladder, 76, 77, 79
calories
per gram, 76
sources, 69
calorie-weight connection,
74
Camellia sinensis, 90, 91–92
Canadian bacon, 111–112

canned food
pumpkin, 129
soup, 128–129
tomatoes, 129
tuna, 129
wild salmon, 130
canola oil, 133–134
carbohydrates, 44, 46
catechin polyphenol, 91
cellular respiration, 44
cellulose, 28–29
cereal, 53, 130–131
cheating, 9–13
cheese, 34, 110, 119–120,
206–207
chickpeas, 54
chicory root, 132
chlorine, 31, 38
chocolate, 39–42
cholesterol, and fat, 59
cis double bond, 62
clothing, 100
coconut extract, 137
coffee, 89–96
coleslaw dressing, 135
complex carbohydrate, 28,
44, 46
condiments, 135–138
cooking oils, 133–134
cooking sprays, 134
corn puffs, 130
Cosi, 173
cow's milk, 116
crackers, 22–23, 45
cravings, sweets, 39
cream, 117
cream cheese, 120
creamy snacks, 207–208

crispbreads, 23, 138, 151
cyanide, 10

D
dairy, 34–36, 116–121
    milk, cream, 116–117
    and saturated fat, 66
dehydration, 89–90
deli, 110
desserts, 39–42, 126–127
diabetes, 59, 95
diet industry, 12
dinner
    and calorie ladder, 78
    menus, 78–204
dips, 110, 119
distraction, and coffee, 90–92
"the dose makes the poison,"
    9–11, 40
double bonds, 61–62
dried fruits, 20–21
drinks, 38–39
dry foods, 16, 18
durum wheat semolina, 140

E
ectomorphic, 45
edamame, 110, 126
eggs, 65, 118
electrolytes, and coffee,
    89–90
endomorphic, 45
energy, 44, 45
energy-dense foods, 17
entrees, frozen, 125–126
erythritol, 30, 37, 41, 132
essential fatty acids, 62
expeller-pressed oils, 70–71
extracts, 37, 137
extra virgin olive oil
    (EVOO), 133

F
"fake butter," 71
fast carb, 47–48
fat
    and calories, 68–72
    and carbohydrate, 44
    cells, 58
    dangers of, 58–59
    in foods, 61–63
    and genetics, 57–58

and liver, 58–59
    storage, 57–58, 60
fat-free sour cream, 120
fat-free vinaigrettes, 135
fatty liver disease, 58
FDA, 38
feta cheese, 120
flavored water, 39, 124
flax pasta, 139
flax seeds, 116
FOS (fructooligosaccharides),
    27–28, 29, 37, 41
the "fourth macronutrient,"
    15
fractionated oil, 63
free snacks, 212
freeze-dried fruit, 21, 141
frozen foods, 125–127
frozen waffles, 127
fructo-oligosaccharides.
    see FOS
fructose, 26, 27
fruit, 32–34, 114–115
    bake-dried, 141
    dried, 20–21
    freeze-dried, 141
    freezing, 34
    juice, 33
    limiting, 33
    snacks, 206
    warming, 34

G
galactose, 27
gas, 29–30, 31, 109
gastric bypass procedures, 75
gefilte fish, 130
gelatine, 138
"globesity" epidemic, 17
glucomannan, 140
glucose, 26, 27
glycemic index (GI), 75
glycemic load, 46–47, 75–77
goal weight, 101
gout, and fat, 59
Greek Take-Out, 204, 215
Greek yogurt, 120–121
Green Circle, explained, 148
green tea, 89, 90, 123

H
half and half cream, 117
hangover, 86–87

Health Professionals Follow-
    up Study, 95–96
heart disease, and fat, 60
herbal tea, 91–92
herbs, instead sweetness, 37
The Hershberg Diet, 6, 15
high fructose corn syrup
    (HFCS), 16, 30–31, 41
high glycemic load, 47
high heels, 103
high-water foods, 15–18
hosiery, 102
hot chocolate, 123
hummus, 55, 110
hypoglycemic response, 47

I
infusions (herbal tea), 91–92
insulin resistance, 47
inulin, 28, 48, 140
Italian Take-Out, 187–188

J
Japanese Restaurant Orders,
    193–194
Japanese Take-Out, 187,
    215, 222
jasmine green tea, 123
jerky, 21–22, 141
juice, 124

K
kamut puffs, 130
kidney beans, 54

L
lactose, 26, 27
lap bands, 75
legumes, 54–55
leptin, 16–17
licorice tea, 123
light
    beer, 82
    cheeses, 119–120
    hot chocolate, 123
liquid egg whites, 118
lollipops, 142
low calorie density foods, 17
low-calorie high-water
    foods, 17
low CD foods, 17
low-fat dairy products, 35

low glycemic load, 47
low-water foods, 16
lunch
   and calorie ladder, 78
   menus, 78–204

M
macronutrients, 41, 44
manifesto, 2–3
man-made sugar, 30–31
mannitol, 29
maple syrup, 133
margarine, 118–119
matzos, 23, 138, 151, 217
mayonnaise, 137
meal categories, explained,
   148
measuring tape, 97
meats, 65, 110–112
Mediterranean Take-Out,
   204, 219
Melba toast, 138
meringues, 142
mesomorphic, 45
metabolism, 95
milk, 116–117
milk fat, 34
millet puffs, 130
mirror, 100–103
mitochondria, 74
mixes (alcohol), 82
moderation, 13
monochrome look
   (clothing), 101–102
monounsaturated fat, 62
morbidly obese, 99
mother's milk, 34
mustard, 137

N
National Institute of Health,
   99
neurotransmitters, and
   caffeine, 92
non-dairy cream, 117
"no sugar added," 32
nutrition bars, 143–145
nutritious sugars, 41
nuts, 18–20, 115–116
nutty snacks, 208–209

O
oatmeal, 131
obesity, 12, 17, 99
Okinawa, 17
omega 3
   eggs, 159
   fat, 62
   and unsaturated fat,
      67–68
omega 6 fat, 62
oolong (red) tea, 90, 91
overweight, 99

P
panko breadcrumbs, 109
Paracelsus, 9
partially hydrogenated fat,
   oil, 62–63
pasta, 48–50, 139–141
peanut butter, 20, 136
Penn State, 16
pita, 152, 175–176
pizza, 126
placebo effect, 25
planning, and desserts, 41
polyphenols, 91, 96
polyunsaturated fat, 62
popcorn, 209–210
popsicles, 127
portions, 73–80
potatoes, 51–52, 114
pounds of food per day,
   15, 76
powdered peanut butter,
   20, 136
prebiotic, 48
prepackaged desserts, 40
probiotic, 140
produce, 112–115
protein
   bars, 143–145
   calories per gram, 76–77
   powders, 143
puffed cereals, 53, 130
pumpkin, canned, 129

Q
quinoa, 139

R
rebiana, 30, 132
red wine, 10

restaurant orders, 189
rice, 52, 139
rice puffs, 130
rice wine vinegar, 134
ricotta cheese, 119–120
rooibos tea, 91–92
ruching (clothing), 102

S
salad dressings, 134–135
salads, 178–186
sandwiches, 171–173
saturated fat, 61–66
scale (weight), 97–98
seeds, 18–20, 115–116
Sensato, 30
serving size, 107
sesame oil, 134
75 gram glucose tolerance
   test, 47
shakes, 161–162, 165–166
shelf life, 16, 62
shirataki noodles, 49, 140
shoes, 102–103
simple carbs, 28
simple sugar, 26
small meals v. big meals,
   78–79
smoothies, 161–162, 165–166
snacks, 141–142, 205–212
soda water, 124
sorbitol, 29
soups, 128–129, 173
sour cream, 120
soybean pasta, 139
soy beans, 54
spaghetti squash, 52, 114
Spanx body-shaping
   undergarments, 102
spices, 37, 137
spinach, as carb, 45–46
Splenda, 26, 37–38, 123
spreads, 135–138
squash, 52, 114
Starbucks nutritional
   information, 94
starch, 28–29
stevia, 30, 37, 132
stimulation, and coffee,
   90–92
stomach requirement, 15, 76
stripes (clothing), 102
subcutaneous fat, 57–60

substitutes for sweetness, 37
sucralose, 26, 31, 32, 38
sucrose, 26, 27
sugar
  alcohol, 29, 30
  as building block, 27
  crashes, 47
  molecules, 27
  source, 26
  substitutes, 36–38,
    131–133
  table, 26, 36, 41
  weaning off, 36–37
  withdrawal (hangover), 87
sugar 101, 26–32
"sugar free," 32
sun, 10
supersize, 75
sweeteners, 36–38
sweet potatoes, 51–52, 114
sweet snacks, 209–212

T
table sugar, 26, 36, 41
take-out, 187–188
tea, 89, 90–92, 123
Thai Take-Out, 204
the three Ps, 98
toasted sesame oil, 134
tonic water, 83
toppings, breakfast, 151–152,
    152–153
tortillas, 50–51
toxins
  coffee beans, 96
  hangover, 87
Trader Joes, 106
trans double bond, 62
trans fat, 62–64
trans unsaturated fat, 62
treats, 141–142
trickery, and coffee, 92–93
Truvia, 30, 37
turkey, 46

U
unsaturated fat, 63, 66–68
U.S. Department of
  Agriculture Economics
  Research Service, 31

V
vanilla extract, 137
vegan appetizer, 126
vegetable cocktail, 124
vegetable juice, 124
vegetables, 112–114
vegetarian
  bacon bits, 138
  burgers, 126
Vietnamese Take-Out, 204
vinegars, 134
virgin
  Bloody Mary, 39
  mimosa, 33
visceral fat, 58–60

W
waffles, 127
waistline, and fat, 59
warm snacks, 209
water, 15, 124
water content, 15–16
water-rich foods, 41
weight loss goals, 97–100
Weight Watchers, and trans
  fat, 63
white fat, 57–58
white wine vinegar, 134
Whole Foods, 106
whole wheat high-fiber
  pasta, 49
whole wheat pasta, 139
wine, 82, 84–85
women, and fat, 60
World Health Organization
  (WHO), 17
wraps, 174–175

X
xylitol, 29

Y
yeast, 50
yellow fat, 57, 58, 60
yogurt, 11, 120–121

RECIPES

A
apples, 156, 160–161

B
banana, 161, 166
beans
  chili, 173
  salad, 180
breads
  French toast, 163
  fried matzo, 164
  peanut butter cracker-
    sandwiches, 208
  stuffed pita, 176
broccoli slaw, 207
butternut squash, 198

C
cauliflower, 201
chicken
  Asian salad, 181–182
  Caesar salad, 179–180
  Chicken and Salad,
    189–190
  Crispy Chicken Breasts,
    197–198
  fajitas, 201–202
  Greek salad, 178–179
  grilled, 190
  quesadilla, 190–191
  tenders, 198–199

D
deli sandwich, 171
drinks
  Banana Wake-Up, 161
  Berry Wake-Up, 161
  chocolate banana shake,
    166
  Iced Mocha, 161–162
  Iced Vanilla Rebelccino,
    158
  Orange Dream, 165
  strawberry banana
    shake, 165

E
eggs
 Egg Muffin To Go, 157
 sandwich, 172
 omelets, 154–155, 160

F
fish
 baked, 200
 Fave Fish Dinner, 182
 halibut with rice and
  vegetables, 190
 Manischewitz Gefilte
  Fish, 182
 salmon and salad, 191
 salmon cakes, 193
 salmon noodle salad,
  185–186
 shrimp Greek salad,
  178–179
 stuffed tuna pita, 176–
  177
 tuna and veggie noodle
  salad, 192–193
 tuna noodle salad, 184
 tuna sandwich, 171
French toast, 163
fruit
 banana shake, 161
 berry shake, 161
 chocolate banana shake,
  166
 Orange Pineapple Jell-O
  Dessert, 211
 strawberry banana
  shake, 165

G
guacamole, 196

K
kale, 202
kamut squares, 164

M
matso, 164
muffins, 157

O
omelets, 154–155, 160

P
pasta and noodles
 Asian tilapia on angel
  hair pasta, 184–185
 pasta pPrimavera, 203
 pasta salad, 183
 pesto pasta, 203–204
 shirataki Alfredo, 186
 tuna noodle salad, 184
peanut butter cracker-
 sandwiches, 208–209
pesto, 203–204
potato skins, 199–200
pumpkin cheesecake,
 211–212

S
salads
 Asian chicken, 181
 bean and seed, 180
 Caesar, 179–180
 Cobb, 180–181
 Greek, 178–179
 pasta, 183
 salmon noodle, 185–186
 tuna noodle, 184, 192–
  193
sandwiches and wraps
 chicken, 175–176
 chicken wrap, 175–176
 deli, 171
 egg salad, 171
 havarti, tomato, and
  basil, 195
 homemade chicken
  wrap, 175–176
 stuffed Greek pita, 176
 stuffed tuna pita, 176–
  177
 tuna, 171
snacks
 broccoli slaw, 207
 Jell-O, 211
 peanut butter cracker-
  sandwiches,
  208–209
 pumpkin cheesecake,
  211–212
soups
 French onion, 173–174
 Moroccan lentil, 173
 tomato, 173
spaghetti squash, 1191–192
sweet potato, 183–184, 190

V
vegetables
 broccoli slaw, 207
 butternut squash, 198
 cauliflower, 201
 kale chips, 202
 potato skins, 198–199
 spaghetti squash, 191–
  192
 sweet potato, 183–184,
  190
 zucchini, 199

PRODUCTS

A
A.C. LaRocco Bruchetta Style
 Pizza, 126, 195, 222
All-Bran
 Buds, 130
 Original Cereal, 130,
  154, 164
Allegro 4% Ricotta, 119–120
Amy's Kitchen, 125, 170,
 188, 195
 Apple Toaster Pop, 162,
  220
 Bean & Cheese Burrito,
  218
 Cheese Pizza in a Pocket
  Sandwich, 220
 Cream of Rice Hot
  Cereal Bowl, 162
 Mexican Casserole Bowl,
  214
 Organic Soups, 128–129
 Strawberry Toaster Pop,
  162, 220
 Toaster Pops, 127
Apetina Light feta cheese,
 120
Arrowhead Mills, 130
Astro
 Original Balkan Style
  Natural Yogourt, 36,
  66, 120, 217
 Original Fat Free
  Yogourt, 36, 120
 Original 1% Yogourt,
  120
Au Bon Pain, 173

B

Baked Lay's, 174, 221, 223
Baker's Deluxe High Fibre
    Bagels, 51, 109
BALANCE Bars, 144, 162,
    221
Bare Fruits
    100% Granny Smith
        Apple Chips, 153,
        206, 218
    100% Organic Bake-
        Dried Fuji Apple
        Chips, 141
Becel Light, 118
Becel Topping and Cooking
    Spray, 71, 114, 118–119,
    152–153, 156, 160, 163,
    221
Bell Plantation PB2
    Powdered Peanut Butter.
    see PB2
Blue Diamond Almond
    Breeze, 19, 35, 40,
    116–117
Blue Goose Cattle Company
    Original Beef Jerky,
    22, 141
Bob's Red Mill
    Brownie Mix, 70
    rolled oats, 154
Boca
    Original Chik'n Nuggets,
        126
    Original Patties, 126
    Spicy Chik'n Patties, 126
Breakstone's cottage cheese,
    119, 151, 153, 207
Breyers 100 Calorie Ice
    Cream Cups, 127, 206,
    209, 223
Brothers-All-Natural crisps,
    141

C

Calabro fat-free ricotta
    cheese, 119
Campbell's soups, 129, 173,
    209
Carnation Hot Chocolate
    Light, 123, 209
Catelli pasta, 49, 139
Cheez Whiz Light, 113, 136,
    152, 206, 207, 217–219

Chocolite
    Chocolates, 40
    Finally! bars, 40, 144
    Protein Bars, 144, 153,
        210
Clif 20g Protein Builder's Bar,
    145, 166, 216, 223
Coffee-mate Lite, 94
Cool Whip 95% Fat Free, 63

D

Dairy Queen, 41, 210–211,
    221, 222, 224
Dannon Light & Fit Yogourt
    60 Calorie Packs, 121
Diet Snapple on Ice Pops,
    127, 212
Dimpflmeier Pumpernickel
    Bread, 107, 108, 195
Dixie Diners' Club Sugar
    Not, 132
Doctor's CarbRite Diet Bars,
    144, 162, 210, 221
Dofino Light Havarti Slices,
    110
Dreamfields Pasta, 48, 140,
    203–204

E

e.d. Smith Pure Pumpkin,
    129
Edward and Sons Organic
    Breadcrumbs, 109

F

Fage 0% Total Yogurt,
    120–121
Fiber One cereal, 130–131,
    154
Food for Life
    Ezekial 4:9 Organic
        Sprouted 100%
        Whole Grain
        Flourless Bread,
        107, 195
    Ezekial 4:9 Pocket Bread,
        107
    Ezekial 4:9 Sprouted
        Whole Grain Bread,
        152, 170, 218, 220,
        222

Genesis 1:29 Organic
    Sprouted Grain &
    Seed Bread, 108
Whole Grain Brown Rice
    Tortillas, 109
Frontier Certified Organic
    Bac'Uns, 70, 138
FullBar, 145, 163, 210
Funky Monkey Freeze-Dried
    Fruit, 141

G

Gay Lea Light Spreadables,
    118, 164
Genuine Health proteins+,
    143
GG Scandinavian Bran
    Crispbreads, 23, 138–
    139, 151, 207, 217
Golden Valley Premium
    Natural Turkey Jerky,
    22, 141
Good Earth Sweet & Spicy
    Herbal Tea, 123
Guiltless Gourmet Fat Free
    Black Bean Dip, 55,
    135–136, 208

H

Häagen-Dazs 97% Fat Free
    Sorbet and Yogourt
    bar, 210
Health is Wealth, 125, 126
Healthy 'N Fit 100% Egg
    Protein Powder in
    Heavenly Chocolate, 143
Hint Essence Water, 124
Hormel deli meats, 111, 112
House Foods shirataki
    noodles, 49, 50, 106,
    140–141

I

Ian's Panko Breadcrumbs,
    109
Imagine Organic Soups,
    128, 209

J

Jell-O, 138, 210
Just Like Sugar, 28, 37, 132

K

Kashi GOLEAN, 127, 131
Kavli, 23
  Crispy Thin Crispbreads,
    138, 151, 208, 217
  Multigrain Melba Toast,
    208
Keen's Dry Mustard, 137
Kikkoman
  Instant Miso Soups, 128
  Panko Bread Crumbs,
    109
Knox gelatine, 138
Kraft
  Calorie-Wise Coleslaw
    Dressing, 135
  Fat Free Mayonnaise,
    137
  Light Cheddar, 119
  Light Done Right
    dressings, 135
  Light Smooth Peanut
    Butter, 136
  Part Skim Mozzarella,
    119

L

La Tortilla Factory Multi
  Grain Wrap, 51, 78, 107,
  109, 152, 170, 175, 190
Laughing Cow
  cheese products, 70
  Light Cheese, 52
  Light Gourmet Cheese
    Bites, 152, 155, 156,
    160, 161, 183, 186,
    206, 207
  Light Swiss Original
    Cheese, 119
Lean Cuisine, 125
  Spa Creamy Chicken
    Alfredo, 220
  Spa entrées, 169
  Spa frozen entrées, 188
Libby's 100% Pure Pumpkin,
  129
Lilydale Fully Cooked Sliced
  Chicken Breasts, 110,
  175, 189
Lipton Cup-a-Soup, 128
Lucerne cottage cheese, 119

M

Mama Lupe Tortillas, 109
Manischewitz Gefilte Fish,
  130, 182
Maple Grove Farms salad
  dressings, 134
Maple Leaf Simply Savour
  Grilled Meat Strips, 111
McCann's Irish Oatmeal, 131
McDonald's, 13
  Bacon Ranch Salad, 216
  Breakfast Burrito, 166,
    215
  Egg McMuffin, 166
  Fruit'n Yogurt Parfait,
    162, 206, 216
  Ice Cream Cone, 210
  salads, 177–178, 216
  Snack Wrap, 175, 214
  Sundae, 41, 206
MimicCreme Unsweetened
  Cream Substitute, 117
Mini Babybel Light Cheese,
  70, 119, 157, 206, 214,
  221
Miss Meringue, 142, 209
Multifibre Melba Toast, 23,
  138, 151, 173, 217
Multi-Grain Cheerios, 130,
  154, 165, 217

N

Nature's Own 100% Whole
  Wheat Bread, 108
Nature's Path
  Kamut Puffs, 53, 164,
    210, 214
  Organic Frozen Waffles,
    127, 162, 166, 220
  organic puffed cereals,
    130, 154
Newman's Own
  Natural Salad Mists, 135
  salad dressing, 135, 184,
    216
New Sun cookies, 131, 154,
  210, 215
No Pudge! Original Fat Free
  Fudge Brownie Mix, 70,
  142, 210, 222
Nordica cottage cheese,
  119, 153
NOW Foods Erythritol,
  30, 132

Nutrition Kitchen pasta,
  49, 139

O

O.N.E Coconut Water, 124
Optimum Nutrition 100%
  Whey, 143
Oreo Blizzard, 41, 211, 221
Organic Meadow light cream
  cheese, 120
Orville Redenbacher's 100
  Calorie Mini Bags, 141,
  218
Ovaltine, 39–40

P

PAM, 134
PB2, 20, 136, 152, 159, 221
PC Blue Menu, 39, 125
  deli meats, 111
  dressings, 135
  8-Vegetable Cocktail,
    124
  English muffins, 108
  entrées, 169
  frozen entrées, 195
  Multi-Grain Instant
    Oatmeal, 162
  oatmeal, 131
  Oven Roasted Chicken
    Breast, 189
  Plum Sauce, 125, 137
  Reduced Fat Macaroni &
    3 Cheeses, 220
  Sliced Chicken Breasts,
    110–111
  Soda, 124
  Steel-Cut Oats with Wild
    Blueberries, 127,
    162, 222
  Vegetable Cocktail, 124
Perrier, 38–39, 124
Philadelphia Light Cream
  Cheese, 120
Piller's Tastes Better than
  Bacon, 78, 111, 156, 159
President's Choice
  Imported Meringue
    Nests, 142, 210
  Licorice Spice Herbal
    Tea, 123

Q

Quaker rolled oats, 154

R

Reddi-wip Original Whipped Light Cream, 117–118, 158
Renée's Ravin' Raspberry Dressing, 216
R.W. Knudsen Very Veggie Juice, 124
Ryvita Light Rye Crispbreads, 138, 151, 207, 217

S

Schneiders Canadian Back Bacon, 111–112, 157
Sensato Erythritol Crystals, 132
Sensible Foods
  Crunch Dried Fruit, 53, 141, 153, 206, 210, 217
  100% Organic Apple Harvest, 21
Siso Whey Protein Isolate, 143
Skinny Cow ice creams, 126, 209, 215
Snack'n Go! hummus, 110
So Delicious Dairy Free Minis, 127
SoNu Water, 124
Soup at Hand
  Blended Vegetable Medley, 129
  Garden Tomato, 129
  Half Fat Cream of Mushroom, 129
Spectrum
  Canola Spray Oil, 134
  cooking sprays, 70
Starbucks Perfect Oatmeal, 162, 166
Streits Whole Wheat Matzos, 138
Subway
  Chili, 223
  Mini Sub, 174
  salads, 178, 214, 221
  6 inch sub, 174, 216
Summer Fresh, 110

SweetPerfection, 28, 132
Swiss Chalet, 197
Swiss Miss Diet Hot Cocoa, 123

T

Thomas' Original English Muffins, 108
Tim Hortons
  Chicken Wrap Snacker, 175, 216
  low fat muffin, 166
  Low Fat Yogurt with Berries, 162
Trader Joe's Low Fat Vanilla Yogurt, 121
True Lemon, True Lime, 39, 124
Truvia sweetener, 106, 132
Tyson, 111, 189

V

Van's 97% Fat Free Waffles, 127, 162, 166, 214
V8 Vegetable Cocktail, 39, 124, 156, 157
Vitalicious
  Muffins, 131
  Muffin Tops, 40, 131, 154, 210, 215, 221
Vitamin Water 10, 124

W

Walden Farms
  Calorie Free Apple Butter, 137, 152, 162, 166, 220, 222
  Calorie Free Dressing, 180–181
  Calorie Free Maple Syrup, 38
  Calorie Free Pancake Syrup, 133, 162, 163, 166, 214, 220
Wasa Light Crispbreads, 23, 138, 151, 207, 217
Weight Watchers
  bagels, 109, 195, 208, 223
  English muffins, 108
  snacks, 40

100% Whole Wheat Sliced Bread, 50, 78, 107, 108, 152, 163, 170, 173, 195, 218, 221
Wellshire Organic Turkey Bacon, 111
Wendy's
  Hot Stuffed Baked Potato, 184, 216
  Junior Frosty, 210
Whole Foods
  applesauce, 137
  365 Organic Coffee Creamer Natural Vanilla Flavor, 117
  365 Organic Multi-Grain oatmeal, 131
Wholesome Sweeteners Organic Raw Blue Agave, 132
  Organic Zero, 30, 37, 132, 158
Wonder
  Light Wheat Bread, 108
  Plus English muffins, 108

Y

Yoplait, 38, 121, 154, 207
YummyEarth Organic Lollipops, 142, 210
Yves Veggie Breakfast Links, 157

Z

Ziggy's
  deli meats, 111
  International Havarti Slices, 110